Forged By Fire

By Annie Burns

All rights reserved. No part of this publication may be reproduced or transmitted by any means, including electronic, mechanical, photocopy, or otherwise without the prior permission of the publisher.

For more information, contact: anita.burns@thebluequillstudio.com

First Published in Ontario, Canada in October 2017.

ISBN: 978-0-9949486-0-1

Copyright © The Blue Quill Studio 2017

In dedication to all those who have, or are currently, suffering, or have lost a loved one, due to mental health challenges.

Special thank yous to:
Cassandra Morgan- for being my friend, and writing mentor.
Sammie L. - For your support while trying to make this into a published work.
And, to my beloved sister- I would not be here today if not for her continued love and support

Please Read Before Continuing:

The following is the real thoughts, memories, and opinions of someone with mental health disability. The names of those involved have been changed for the sake of their privacy. There will be will be mature and/or sensitive topics, mild sexual content, and course language.

Reader's discretion is highly advised.

Table of Contents

Welcome to the Forge..1
Miss Piggy...2
My Sister's Charade...4
The Green-Eyed Monster...12
The Nameless Ones..16
Sisters...21
The Hail Mary Pass..29
The Black Sheep...37
5 AM...43
The Step-Father..45
A Sceptical Prophecy...48
Brushes...56
Dig Deep...59
Climbing Everest in the Buff...63
Monsters, Screamers, and Creepers...69
Life Badges..75
Once Terrible Tuesday Morning..78
Hot Tempered and Panicked..86
The Summer of '05..91
To Market..97
Broken-Hearted..102
My Familiars..116
Overcoming Weeds..125
Now Boarding..133
Christmas Lights..144
All You Need is Love..148
Grumbling..151
Don't Touch the Switch...154
Christmas with the Sporidnenyy..157
You Do What You Can..166
Kidlets and Chijens..172
One of Those Moods..175
Mr Boomerang...176
Hope...183
Home For the Holidays..184

Table of Contents

Morning Musings..188
After Christmas Calm-Down..191
Nothing To Prove..193
Melancholy..195
Day One in Pantanal...201
In Case of Emergency...206
Mother Knows Best..210
Unexpected..222
A Waste...225
Fidget...227
The Cardboard Cafe...232
Escape Rooms and Candy Hugs..237
Courage...242
Re-Freed..253
Weakness...258
February 14th..262
You Are Stronger Than This...269
Bonding...274
The Runaway..279
An Idea...282
Living Nightmares..285
Invasion of Privacy...290
Choices..294
The Dragon Egg...296
Making A Comeback..300
Paper Cranes..301
Fixing A Broken Lamp...308
What Happiness Feels Like..311
Healthy Changes..318
Goodbye, Mr Shepard..322
Carpe Diem...323

Welcome to the Forge

Drowning. Too often, this is the word used to describe what depression feels like. I can see why such a metaphor is used. You work your hardest to keep your head above water, while the waves and the undertow attempt to drag you down into darkness.

I hate that metaphor.

For all it's truths, I prefer to think of depression like burning alive. It's painful, and though you scream with all your might, you feel like no one hears you. You're isolated, slowing being burned away into something you don't recognize.

You become chocked into silence by the smoke, better known as insecurity, self-loathing, and social pressure.

Drowning gives hope. Hope that you might be plucked from the sea if you just tread hard enough. That, eventually, you'll be able to put the experience behind you and sail forward toward your dreams.

I haven't known that to be true. The scars are still there. They're only seen by those who know the fire themselves; those who have survived.

You battle with your own mind and hope these are just trials and tests to forge you into something greater than you currently are. Shining, cold metal, or fragile glass art. Either way, you won't be even remotely close to what you once were. The likelihood is, you might not ever escape the flame. You lie to yourself, because it's easier than admitting you're burning away to nothing.

It can be beaten, however.

My name is Annie. This is my inner fire, and how I work to overcome it.

Miss Piggy

I'm sitting naked in front of my laptop.

Don't try to picture that.

I am trying to summon the will to make myself something to eat. I've only eaten a bowl of cereal in the last twenty hours. My stomach is grumbling, but I have no interest in standing in my kitchen to cook. I can hear my mother's voice in my head, telling me I'm just being lazy. Funny that I haven't lived with her for two years, and I still hear the cutting remarks that she's not there to make.

Like remarks concerning my hygiene. Truth be told, I hate feeling dirty and sweaty. I don't know why I see something as simple as a daily shower as such a chore. I love the feeling of being clean, and smelling of whatever new shower gels I've picked up. Tahiti Dream is my current obsession.

I know people can see I haven't bathed in days. Though, with how often I leave my new home these days, it's rare people see me at all. But when they do, I know they notice my grease slicked hair and oily skin. Right now, it's just me, my two cats, and my mother's voice.

"Don't be so lazy," it repeats. "You need to take more pride in your appearance." My appearance means a lot to her.

I remember the time we were in her van, and she felt the need to point out I've gained weight.

"I'm not saying it to be offensive!" she would cover.

How is bluntly saying, "I've noticed your putting on a little weight" not supposed to be offensive? I have a thousand and one other mental tortures to work through in a day. The fact that I'm obese is the least of my concerns right now. Five foot six inches, and 270 lbs. I have always been overweight, and I'm comfortable enough in my skin to be nude.

What bothers me is that my fat ass apparently bothers her. As if me losing a hundred pounds would suddenly get me friends and catch a man's interest so that I'm not alone. It probably would. The people that judge according to one's body are not the kind of people I want to be around, though.

But it doesn't seem to matter to my mother who I am around. Only that there are people around at all.

There it is. The familiar heat of self-loathing coursing through my veins. I'm judging myself from my grease laden hair slicked to my head, to the three days worth of chores piling up around me.

At least I finally have the will to go clean myself. Tahiti Dream is calling my name.

My Sister's Charade

It's Monday. I was supposed to attend my 2D and 3D media class. I ended up sleeping until 2:30 pm instead. I would have slept longer if my cat had not woken me.

So, here I sit. It's 4:00 PM, and I just want to go back to bed. The sad thing is, as soon as I woke up, I wanted to jump onto my laptop, and do my next passage. I'm not sure why this is so addictive. I had to force myself to have some cereal, and attempt to do something with my day. I ended up watching YouTube videos, and venturing through old files to see what I could delete to make space.

I ended up coming upon one that I had not looked at in some time. When I was younger, I used to write letters to my mother when she upset me, and I couldn't handle it anymore. I am not, nor have I ever been, capable of voicing my distress. Especially in the wake of my mother's ire. I would leave copies out for her to find, but too many times of her spreading what was meant to be a discussion opening to everyone that would listen (and dismissing the point while she was at it), it became too much a hassle to continue.

It didn't stop the letters. I wrote them as if she would read them to avoid bottling everything inside. It just stopped me from sending them. I dated each document and buried them into a file folder. A folder I found through my perusing. I'm sorely tempted to read them.

On the one side, I may feel better knowing that something that had upset me before, doesn't bother me now. The problem is, there are a lot of things that bother me now. My family members and I are not very good at giving apologies. Usually, the guilty starts to treat the other as if nothing had happened, until the other person does the same. That is our apology, and forgiveness.

Except, we don't forgive. Not really. Because we were never sorry.

It's November, and I'm still bristling about the way my mother handled my sister, Camilla, and mine's birthdays. The good side is, I'll still be angry when March rolls around. I will be ready, this year, when my sister continues her charade that she's mad at me for one thing or another. That way she can't point at me, and cry, "she ruined my birthday!" And then everyone will go out of their way to make it better. She's been doing it for a couple of years now. Every year, however, I have put the little stunt behind me. Only, I end up forgetting that she does it until I've already fallen into it again. Not this year, though.

See, this time, my sister had invited me to go to a party thrown by people I thought were mutual friends. Not all of them, mind you, but there were a couple. Such as Kevin, my oldest friend from our days back in elementary school. I'm the reason he and my sister know one another. Apparently, that doesn't mean a damn thing.

I went for the sake of socializing. I had been unemployed for so long, and left alone in my apartment for days or even weeks at a time, that my depression was getting worse. Too much time to over-think and worry about where the next meal was coming from. At the time, I did not have any official diagnosis about mental health. Cam thought she was being nice by bringing me to be around her friends.

The thing is, I don't drink. I don't like loud music, especially the kind my sister and these guys seem to like. It certainly was not the setting for me. Still, I'm an incredibly friendly individual, and fairly good at hiding my anxiety. Most people are none the wiser about my inner fire when they first meet me.

It was a small group of people, and I knew all of them from the local comic store, the GME. It was easy to get into the games, or just sit and listen while we chatted around a fire. I had come up with a King's Cup rule that had people's jaws on the floor.

When I do choose to drink, it would surprise people I have such a high tolerance. Once I start to feel a little warm, I pretend I'm fully drunk. Not the wild and crazy, "Look at me!" sort of drunk. I know to increase my volume, let the vulgarities go, and then I just let myself show how tired I am. Being tired is just a side effect of my mental health combined with the alcohol; even in small amounts. I'm sure to some degree I am intoxicated, but not nearly as much as I lead people to believe that I am.

The reason I do this is because, one, people don't question it as much when I switch to water or pop, and, two, a lot of people find it hilarious.

"Oh look! The prude is drunk!"

Alcohol also has this funny effect on me where I'm not as scatter-brained. I'm less distracted and more focused. Maybe it just eliminates my stress, or counters some chemical imbalance. I don't really drink, so I don't actually know.

What I do know is that I had a lot of fun that night. As did the guys. Most of them are easy enough to understand when they're not drunk, but add a little inebriation, and you can pinpoint who is feeling what. My only fault was that I was paying attention to the guys, and not my sister.

When she had to leave early because Grandpa would stay up until she got home, I did not go with her. I lived on my own and was unemployed. I could stay for as long as Tony, our host, would allow. He, Justin, and I had already set up a tent in the backyard that I had intended to sleep in. It was only then I realized my sister was upset.

At the time, I thought she was jealous that I got to stay and she didn't. After at night, however, I realized what she had been trying to do: make herself look cool in contrast to me. Not only had it blown up in her face, but I had poked fun at her just as many times as she was doing so to me.

There was a week between the night of the party, and my sister's actual birthday of the 14th. Cam is not one to hold back her thoughts. There were plenty of occasions she could have spoke her mind. Including when Sandra had asked how the party went, and I openly told her. But she waited until 10:00 PM on the 13th. Then she let me have it.

She started a fight with me through Facebook Messenger. She went on and on about how I embarrassed her and made the party awkward for everyone. What nerve I had to ruin HER birthday party, in front of HER friends, when she was kind enough to bring me out to socialize. During her rant, she made it sound like I should worship her for her 'kindness'.

What she did not know was that I was not at home that night. I was dog-sitting for Mum until she was done at work at 10:30 pm. I ended up staying the night because I figured I would go with Mum to see my sister for her birthday. Mum said she would take me to get cat litter, as well, since she had her own errands to do.

When Mum got home, I immediately told her that Cam decided to start a fight. For once, I had the proof. I didn't say as much, but I was ecstatic when my mother responded with, "You noticed you two are always in a fight on her birthday, and it's supposedly your fault?"

At last, my mother could see for herself what my sister was doing. Cam was not going to get away with it. Even if my grandmother was babying my sister- which she would, because my grandmother openly picks favourites- Mum knew the truth. I figured the 14th was going to proceed as originally planned. Sure, my sister would be pissed off, but maybe next year she wouldn't pull the same shit.

Except she did get away with it.

My Mum had to work the next morning, until 2:30 PM. While I was set and ready to go, she did not come home until a little over two hours later. Why? Because she went to see my sister without me.

My mother is a PSW nurse, that works two jobs. Two hours of her spare time is worth gold to her, and she spent that time with my sister. It was my sister's birthday, so fine. Mum goes to her next client care from 5-6, and after that, we go for our errands. During this time, she insists we hurry because Cam wanted to go to the movies that night.

The way it was said, I already knew I was not invited. I still held out for the benefit of the doubt. Maybe this was how Mum was going to make it clear to my sister she can't treat me this way just so she can be treated special for her birthday.

Except I got dropped off at home.

Mum was trying to tell me that I probably didn't want to be around Cam right now, anyway. I blocked the majority of it out because I was seeing red and turning green. My sister got two hours of my mother's time, AND got to go to the movies without me after starting shit, AGAIN. After the way Cam's birthday went, I was fuming. The words "Fucking spoiled brat" was a common mental phrase for at least a month after that.

I was pissed and tired of my sister's shit. As I collected my bag of cat litter, my Mum looked at me, and said, "Don't let it get-."

But I cut her off, "Too Late!" Then I proceeded to slam the door, and march inside my apartment complex. I figured Mum was going to call and tell me off about my temper tantrum. She did call, but to invite me to go for breakfast.

"No, thanks." I told her, with a tone that was clear I knew this was her trying to make it up to me. I hadn't just spent another day alone - watching my mother's animals for her, at that. I got to deal with the mental ramifications of my sister's actions.

She doesn't care about you. She doesn't even want you around to celebrate her special day. Maybe you really do ruin her birthday. Just like you ruin everything else. You're such a failure at everything. Of course they would dote on Cam while you're always alone. You were the accident child, after all. She was the one Mum wanted to have.

So, yeah, I was not in the mood for Mum's pity, or her little truce gesture.

"I'm not doing this because of today," she pressed. "I want to go for breakfast tomorrow."

I had to laugh at her stubbornness, and agreed to go. I did not sleep well that night. It had been too obvious that I had been crying most of the night. It was this gnawing feeling of loneliness that stemmed from the idea that, of the people my sister wants to celebrate her existence with, I was not one of them. And our family was okay with that. Mum, thankfully, did not bring attention to how much I looked like Hell had thawed over the next morning.

Not until breakfast had arrived, at least. I think she thought if she approached the topic before that, I would have stormed out. Now I was obligated to sit there and eat my meal that she had been gracious enough to buy for me. Honestly, I don't think I would have had the energy. Plus, I knew, though I was miffed at Mum for how she handled my sister's actions, my true anger was at Cam. There was no point having a fit at the wrong person, and I was just glad it was a new day.

She repeated the things she had said on the night before my sister's birthday. All the things that was done as part of treating Cam special, and how could Cam treat her own sister that way. I don't think I was commenting enough because Mum paused at one point.

"Well, we'll just have to do something without her for your birthday," she finally stated matter-of-fact.

I smirked, "I'm not that petty."

Because I felt like it was true. June was three months away. That's a long time to hold a grudge, for me. I see no reason to stay angry that long over something that amounted to nothing. There's plenty of other, worse reasons to be upset. I don't need to compound my problems. Besides, I was already letting it go by that morning. I had chalked it up to my sister being herself, and things would go back to normal now that she got what she wanted. She might even do something nice, like send me a funny video or meme on Facebook.

Except that was not the end of it. Where I may not be the type that holds pointless grudges for long, my sister is. I had stood up for myself, and let Mum in on what she was doing. I have no doubt Mum had said something to her at some point about it. Since she already had the charade going to explain "why" she was upset with me, it was easy enough to continue.

I showed up at the GME on Wednesday, thinking we and our friends were going to chat, and might even play a board game. Saturdays are board game days. Wednesdays and Fridays are for Magic the Gathering. Except Wednesdays are far more casual, so it quickly becomes an open night.

I got there, and was immediately given the cold shoulder from my sister. I inwardly rolled my eyes, and went to chat with the guys. Only to be ignored, completely. Kevin was the only one to say hello.

Guess they were just HER friends, after all.

I marched myself home, and forced back the tears on the way. By the time I reached my apartment door, my blood was boiling. I get that they were trying to support her. They're good people like that. It was my sister once again stabbing me in the back.

I texted my mother: "For my birthday, can you and I go somewhere overnight? Just us?"

I figured that was what she was doing for Cam's birthday. A couple weeks later, mind you, because Cam wanted to attend her school open house. It wouldn't be a far stretch to do the same.

Mum called me. She told me she already had June 19th off, so she could arrange a switch for the morning of the 20th. I let it go. Mum and I had our plan, and I figured she would stick to it. I had a plan to make my birthday special while simultaneously giving Cam a minor taste of what exclusion feels like. I didn't even have to start a bullshit fight with my sister to get it. A month later, though, it became clear that I should have.

The Green-Eyed Monster

I know I will eventually tell the other half of the story, but it's not good to dwell in a place of anger. I told myself to calm down, first, and then continue my next passage. Something happy. It's just... I don't want to talk about something happy.

Honestly, I'm tired of burying things. I know that's why I started this. I know that's why I write it as if a stranger was reading it. I'm tired, and I just want someone to see me. Maybe not in a grand way, but just something to make someone happy that I exist.

It's why this birthday stuff bothers me. On the one hand, my sister is waited on daily by our grandparents. Mostly my grandmother. If we wanted to visit, it had to be Cam that asked because I always got a no.

"Look how well Cam dances." So I chose to sit and sing along instead. I still don't dance, now that I think about it.

"Oh, Camilla is so funny!" I often wonder if people actually find me funny, or if I'm just fooling myself.

The only time Cam was not the favourite was after our cousin, Sonia was born. My grandmother always picks the youngest.

I, being the eldest grandchild, never stood a chance at being on my grandmother's radar.

It's probably why I spoil Sonia more than her younger brother, Dean. The poor girl has no idea the reason Grandma pays so much attention to her brother over her, is because that's how Grandma is.

Where my grandmother is blatant about it, my mother insists that she is not doing the exact same thing.

I wasn't allowed to go to camp until my sister was old enough to go too. Never mind that I would eventually be too old to go, giving Cam an extra couple of years without me.

When I was in grade 10, I was regularly seeing my school counsellor. I decided I needed to convince my mother that, yes, I needed help. I snuck behind her back to see a doctor, and when the doctor told me I had mild depression, I called my mother to come talk to this professional.

The result was one week of grounding. I can still hear my mother's reasoning. "I'm not grounding you because you went looking for help, but because you went behind my back. All they're going to do is put you on medication. I could have told you it's just winter blues. Trust me, you'll feel better in the spring."

I didn't end up feeling better. Within a year later, my mother is driving my sister to weekly counselling appointments for depression - in between her guitar lessons. I didn't get lessons, but I did get a self-teaching keyboard. I can learn forty-nine different songs from it. Nothing past that, because I don't know how to read notes.

Right, so now I'm berating myself for bringing up the music lessons. That was a long time ago. It's not even something that bothers me anymore, yet, apparently, it does. Not for what it was, but because its inequality. I have to stop a moment and remember there are two huge things my mother did for me, and not my sister.

Because I was the older one, I got to be an exchange student first. Sure, I spent a few years working my mother down to the idea, but I did get to go to Brazil for seven months. The only reason Cam didn't get to do exchange was because a lot of things went wrong for me while I was there. To shorten a long story, I came home early. I stayed seven months, but I was supposed to be there for ten.

Mum paid for Cam to go on a two-week music trip to Montreal with our high school choir instead. When she's feeling particularly spiteful, my sister tends to bring up how unfair that was. I know it was just Mum trying to protect her from going through the same crap I did.

The other was our trip to Disney World. Mum and Aunt Heather had been planning it for some time, but then Cam ran away from home. She was sixteen, and going through a phase. So, the final deposit was made for two adults, instead of three. Cam finally came home about a month or two before we went. She had been living with my grandparents since she could not be trusted to live at home.

Now, see, that was another thing with Mum. Sixteen-year-old sister puts her through what she did, and is forgiven. Mum and I are starting to get at one another's throats, and I decided, at twenty-three, I should move out. She acts like I was the scum of the earth that had just slapped her.

If it wasn't for my Aunt's help, I wouldn't have been able to even get my first apartment. Heather was the one that came to look at places with me, and then acted as witness when signing my lease. Mum did not visit. I later found out she was telling the family not to visit me either - so that I could "settle in". Further more, she insisted that absolutely nothing of mine was allowed to stay in her house as of my moving day.

Seriously, it was a stressful mess, and she hardly talked to me for two months after the fact. The only messages or words I got from her was over making sure I paid my phone bill.

My sister plans to get her own place in the coming new year. While I was visiting Chatham, the two of them were talking it through. Mum happily providing my sister with advice.

Honestly, my relationship with my mother is freaking complicated.

You know, it's nice to be writing this all out. I know I'm being utterly petty, childish, and angry right now. I know that the deeper I get into things, and the more I unburden what's been left to rot in my soul for so long, the better I'll feel.

In short, I'm going to keep striking nerves. I'm going to be sad. I'm going to be angry. I'm going to paint people in terrible lighting, whether they deserve it or not. I need to keep doing this. I feel like it's making a difference. I need to learn to let myself feel, so I can understand what it is I'm feeling. It's a dangerous thing. I hate how angry I feel. I hate what anger does to people.

But that's just another part of the utterly chaotic mess that fuels my mental fire. For this passage, I'm allowed to be jealous of how my family treats my sister vs me. I'm allowed to feel, I suppose, triumphant, that there are times, though rare, that cause my sister to taste jealousy as well. Still, this gives me a sickly feeling. In the interest of not causing damage when what I'm trying to do is heal, I think I need to go do something else for a little while.

The Nameless Ones

The "something else" I did was go to the store that's down the road from me. I'm not sure why I felt the need to get a 2L pop, but that's what coxed me out of my apartment. I made it there, discovered there was a sale of 4/$5, and then lugged them and the blueberries I also bought, home. Only, when I got home I realized my student card was missing.

Possibly loosing my student card/ bus pass was one stress. I had tucked the little papers with notes about my next appointments in the sleeve the card came with.

I felt uneasy when I emptied my pockets, and discovered it wasn't there. I searched the spots where I would normally put it, and a couple that I wouldn't. Nothing.

I took off back to the store. I figured it must have fallen out when my wallet had dropped out of my pocket during check out. Damn shallow pockets. I made it all the way there, praying the entire time that it could be found. Nothing

The woman behind the check-out had another customer, so I asked the two other employees if I could leave my name with them in case it turns up. The gentleman of the two agreed, and lead me to the back.

"Are you alright?" he asked just as we were turning into the hall to the back.

"Not really." I'm not shy about what I'm feeling. The phrase, 'I'm fine' is too dangerous to utter because, eventually, you start to believe it yourself. The second part was a lie, though. "It just hasn't been a good day for me." In truth, today has been one of my better days in a long time.

The man at the store – Mike, according to his name tag - knew that a student card is also a bus card. He offered me two of his bus tickets. I was beyond shocked by his kindness. I'm still flabbergast. I'll be returning the tickets to him inside a thank you card, now that I've found my student card. The damned thing was on my bed, of all places.

As I walked home, I couldn't help but think how best to thank this kind gentleman. It wasn't just the tickets. He didn't just write my name down, and tell me he'd call if they find it. He looked at me, and talked to me about what I could do if I don't find the card. I hardly spoke, yet, it's like he sensed I needed a plan of action, or else I'd start to panic. This stranger took time out of his day to help this frazzled woman regain some amount of calm and hope.

The saddest part is that no one will know just how much he did for me. Either of us could tell people about the encounter, but it will eventually just fade away from memory. This everyday hero would never receive any worldly recognition. I can hardly remember his face because I was trying to not make eye contact - I have a hard time holding eye contact when I'm upset. I had to write it down, because I don't want to forget this man's kindness.

Truly, God bless him. God bless all those who are selfless and kind, like him.

There were a few people, all nameless, that I can pinpoint in my collected memory that had been kind. A few years back, my mother, sister, and I had driven to Tobermory for our family vacation. We stayed at a campground that was a short drive from the actual town. We had planned on doing the glass bottom boat, and rose early in the morning to take turns at the public shower.

Two factors were at work that morning. The first is that I am not a morning person. Far from it. If I need to be somewhere, I have to set my alarm at least an hour and a half earlier than I need. I can get ready for the day in 20 minutes once I'm actually moving, but getting moving is the issue.

The second is that I have always been rather absent minded, and that's while I'm alert. For some reason, I spent most of my younger years forgetting to grab a towel before hopping into the shower. At home, that meant yelling for a family member to go into the linen closet in the hall, and bring me one. Or march the cold walk, if I was alone.

As you have probably added up, yes, I did forget to grab a towel before going to the showers. Mum and Cam had already had theirs, so they were not coming. There I stood, soaking wet, and cursing myself for being so forgetful. Then, the shower next to mine turned off.

For five minutes, I gently called out to the stranger in the next shower. She did not answer. When I heard her place her bag on the counter, I peaked out to see why she didn't answer. Turns out, it was a little ol' grandmother that was mostly deaf (she had put her hearing aid back in when she noticed me). She later said that my face peeking out of the curtain had spooked her. Better yet, I'm fairly certain her first language was French. Even so, mostly hidden behind a shower curtain, I was somehow able to communicate with her my site number, and that I needed my mum to bring me a towel.

I was not allowed to live that down for several weeks. It was even funnier when we ended up running into her and her family in the line up for the glass-bottom boat. As embarrassing as it was, I am still grateful to that woman. She could have left me there until I either dripped dry, or my mother came to check what was taking me so long. She could have told me to wait until she was finished getting ready. She had no issue trusting me to look after her things while she hurried to get Mum. I actually think of her every time I forget a towel. Yes, that still happens to this day. Thankfully, my current home has a closet in the bathroom.

I remember another senior that had helped me. I don't know who he is, or if he is still alive. I remember I was very small. I don't know how little. In my memory, I'm staring down an escalator, and then back away from it. Then I feel a tight hold on my shoulder, and I'm ushered onto the escalator. For the longest time, I thought I was remembering Mum grabbing me. There was a conversation that led to Mum telling me that it wasn't her. I had been too scared to get on with her.

She couldn't go back up - I think it was something to do with my sister - and was yelling for me to just get on and come down. She told me that it was an old man that had grabbed me by my coat, plunked me on the escalator, and road down with me so that I wouldn't be scared. I don't know who he was, but God, bless him.

The last that comes to mind, was a girl at my high school. I was hidden away in the bathroom that day. I have no idea what it was I was crying about that time. I had not expected anyone to walk in, since it was the middle of first period. I had to be in grade 9 or 10.

When I heard the door creak open, I tried to muffle my sniffles, and just wait until she left. I can still see her black shoes under the stall door as she softly knocked.

"Is everything okay?"

I was unable to answer with words, so I responded with a weak, "mmhmm".

"Are you sure?"

This time I squeaked out a "yes".

She was quiet a moment, and I thought she would leave. Instead, she encourage me to come out. I don't remember the exact words, but it had been enough to get me to unlock the door, and step out. She offered me a kind smile, and a hug. I ended up clinging to her as if my life depended on it. It wasn't a long hug, because I was worried big me would crush her from holding on so tight. She was slightly taller than me, with dark hair, and not a scrap of meat to her.

Still, she smiled, fetched some paper towels, and asked who my teacher was. When I told her, she asked if I wanted her to go get her. I agreed. I let her lead me from the bathroom, and stop in front of my classroom door. There was, mercifully, no one in the hall. She waved down my teacher, so that I didn't have to face my classmates with tear streaks and rosy cheeks. The teacher ended up dismissing me from class so that I could go to the guidance counsellor's office.

I don't remember ever getting the girl's name. I know that once the teacher spoke with me, and decided I should see a counsellor, the girl had to return to class. She gave me another hug before leaving. This one was as tight as the one I had given her in the bathroom.

"You have a pretty smile," she had whispered while we hugged. I'm not sure when I had smiled throughout the meeting.

I had never run into her, again. I mean, our high school was made up of three buildings, and approximately 1700 students. I had kept an eye out in the hallway each time I left my first period that semester. I wanted to thank her, again. A childish side of me wants to think that maybe she was an angel sent to help me, and then had to go help others. Sadly, this is the first time I've thought about her since that year.

Has it already been eleven years? Yeah, I would have been fourteen or fifteen, then. Funny that she is popping into my head now. I wish I knew who she was. Somehow I feel like that moment was one of my darkest hours. Maybe it just felt different because someone heard my soul screaming and did what she could to help. It was not much, but what she did made a difference. For all I know, I may still be here today because she cared enough to knock on the door, and not walk away.

I hope that, whoever and wherever she is, she's happy. All of them. I wish them the best. Those are the kinds of souls that make it easier to face my mental health one day at a time. Funny enough, they always come at the most perfect time.

I guess this passage is a reminder to be kind to others. You never know how much those small actions can make a difference. Whether its a pair of bus tickets, fetching a forgotten towel, or a smile and a hug. Truly, it goes a long way.

Sisters

I've been thinking a lot about my sister.

I know the couple of the times I have mention her, it is when I'm angry or jealous. I don't think that's fair to her. That's why writing this passage felt important.

First of all, when we got older, we did go through a phase of hitting one another. Scraps and flared tempers. Majority of the time she would start it.

That doesn't mean it was solely my sister who would attack first. I used to rough house a lot while growing up. Which meant there were a lot of times I would randomly push, kick, or hit. Most of the time I was gentle. The contact was to be annoying, but not to hurt.

Yet, there were a handful of times that I got pretty brutal.

The first was one night while we were watching TV. I can still remember my sister innocently sitting on the floor. She was actually fairly close to the bulky, heavy TV Mum had owned for as long as I could remember. The basement (which was used like a den/living room) was dark, leaving only the screen as light.

I'm guessing I was about twelve-years-old at the time. Maybe even thirteen. I know I was really into the show we were watching when I was in grades 7 and 8.

I remember going up behind my sister, and then *wham*. One solid, open-handed smack to her back. Younger me thought I was just messing around until Cam regained her wind, and screamed. It was that awful crying-scream that only happens when someone has been seriously injured. Just thinking about it still makes my stomach drop.

The attack had left a perfect red hand-print. My mother had been on the top floor. She said she had clearly heard the *thud* when my hand made contact. Needless to say, I was in some serious shit for it, but I fully deserved it. I don't remember hitting anyone again until our fight when she was sixteen.

Actually, come to think of it, this would have happened

before my fight with Courtney.

Sorry, to put that into context, Courtney was a girl that used to bully me in elementary school.

I didn't know her on a personal level. She was a year younger than me, and had been part of the students transferred to our school after theirs was shut down.

What I did know was that she was the third strongest kid in school. Strongest of the girls, for sure. I can remember thinking that all I needed to do was stand up to her. Use my words. I had hit puberty much earlier than my school mates, so I was larger than her. It was about intimidation. Problem was, Courtney was not the type to be intimidated.

I went up to her, and told her off. I don't know if it was because I snapped, or if I was trying to be touch in front of my sister. Courtney laughed, and taunted me with the classic, "what are you going to do about it,..." She finished off with a name the bullies had given me. I may touch on that another time.

The point is, I had slapped her. I wish I could say I clocked her a good one, but I didn't. As soon as I felt my hand start to swing, my senses jolted into overdrive. Reason shouted at me that this was not how I did things. I pulled the majority of my strength at last minute. The result was a pitiful, four finger tap on her cheek.

She was momentarily surprised that I had attempted to defend myself. Then, her eyes turned steel, and she grabbed the front of my jacket. I was given three hard jabs to my gut. I think my pudgy figure had helped me out that day, because it only hurt until bedtime. After she punched me, she threw me to the ground.

Everything from there is foggy. I assume the years are playing on my memory. I don't remember if anything else was said. I do remember getting up, though. I remember someone grabbing onto my arm as I held Courtney in my sights. My vision was blurred with tears. I know she and her friends left the scene before we did, but I'm not really sure how I got home. I assume we had walked, as the plan had always been.

I know Cam and our friend had to explain what happened. I couldn't put two words together if I tried. Mum had praised me for standing up for myself. The next school day after, there seemed to be a new respect for me among my peers. No one was saying that name anymore. The teasing had cut back to mild annoyances from only a minor handful of people. Most notably, Courtney had stayed far away from me.

It would make sense that I would have pulled back out of fear. After hitting Cam like I had, I knew I would have done some serious damage.

Huh. That was just an interesting train of thought.

Anyway, the other time I attacked first was during recess at our elementary school. I was definitely in grade 8 then. I was about to get into how I know it was that year, but I just realized to explain that would require me to explain about the group I hung out with from the 5th to 8th grade. I've already gone off topic enough this passage. Another passage, perhaps.

Cam and I were having one of our arguments in front of our group of friends. I have no clue what the fight was about. Eventually, she came up, and shoved me. I grabbed her, threw her to the ground, and then sat on her. Not with my full weight, because I didn't want to crush her, but still enough. I can still hear myself cruelly shouting, "this is where you belong. Under me!"

Talk about taking sibling rivalry too far.

That's the only ones that I can remember. I'm sure if I asked my sister, she would list off a thousand others (same as I come out with stuff about her). It's a wonder the two of us even get along with how we treated one another. Granted, I've heard of other people and their siblings doing far worse to one another.

I suppose there are also times we would purposefully get one another into trouble. The earliest example I can remember of that was a long time ago. This was after my mother was separated from Richard, my biological father. Back when we still lived in the Geared-to-income before moving in with Nicholas, my temporary step-father.

This one is super foggy. I remember more of bits and pieces.

We owned a mini-trampoline. It was tiny, but it was big enough for a single child to use. My sister was at an age that she was only just learning to write letters. It left her alphabet very distinctive verse my school-aged scribbles. I ended up taking some crayons, and writing her initial in her style of writing over most of the trampoline. Then I tattled.

Yeah, I was sort of a little shit while growing up.

Don't worry, I did eventually feel guilty, and confess. Still, that was only after my sister had already been punished for something she had not done.

I cut her bangs before picture day once, as well. I don't remember that one at all, but Mum tells the story a lot. She says it was a perfect square. Like I had just grabbed a couple strands, and snipped.

"You couldn't have done it any other day of the year, or on your dolls. Nope, let's cut your sister's hair," she always laughs.

Apparently, she had to comb Cam's bangs a certain way to avoid it showing in the picture. It still sort of does though, if you know what you're looking for.

Oh, I just remembered the time Cam and I were eating breakfast at Nicholas' house. It was a weekend because his two boys were there. We always sat in the same spots at the table. I was on the long side with my back against the wall. Cody, Nicholas' youngest, was to my left, James, Nicholas' oldest, was to the right, and Cam was across from me.

That morning, Cam and I were bickering about which of us was going to marry James one day. The boy in question just looked horrified. I still vaguely recall Nicholas trying to explain to us that neither of us could not marry James because he was our brother. Well, step-brother.

Funnier than that was the time Cam, Mum, and I went to

Point Pelee for a day trip. We were having a good time that the pair of us were super hyper. I could not tell you how many times Mum was rolling her eyes at our antics. She should have saved them to do all at once when we finally reached the Centre. We were waiting for the bus to the point (The most Southern point in all of Canada) when I had spotted the kid's section.

Along the one wall was a bunch of simple kid's costumes. Some of them, like the bat, cactus, and butterfly, fit us. Sort of. Considering I was a plump teenager, that's saying something. There's actually several pictures of us wearing these costumes. Also, despite there not being a costume of one, we suddenly burst out singing, and doing the dance for the camp song, "brown squirrel". I know there's a couple version of the song, but the one Cam and I know goes:

Brown squirrel, brown squirrel, shake your bushy tail!
Brown squirrel, brown squirrel, shake your bushy tail!
Put a peanut in your paw,
and SHOVE-IT UP YOUR NOSE!
Brown squirrel, brown squirrel, shake your bushy tail!

The entire time we had Mum, and the reception lady, in stitches. It only got better when, in the middle of our show, a family with a daughter (maybe seven or eight-years-old) walked into the Centre. The little girl was so excited that she had to come up to say she knew the song too. Thus, we did it again so that she could join us. Granted, she didn't grab a costume.

You know, Cam and I were talking recently, and she reminded me of something I had temporarily forgotten about. While living at Nicholas', we had a pop-up trailer. It never left the drive-way, but the four of us kids were in it all the time. We considered it our secret base, and would pretend to be super spys watching the adults. All four of us were heart-broken the day it was sold.

Now, for the memory that brought up this passage. I was

searching for Christmas cards, but I found two birthday ones that were just too perfect.

The one Cam is going to get reads, "Sister, on you're birthday you deserve to be treated like a Queen" and then on the inside reads, "because you're already a royal pain."

I think the other one was funnier, but I doubt Cam would feel the same. That card has a picture of a cat with it's paws on the keyboard. On the front is, "Dang it... another typo. Dang it... ANOTHER typo."

Then, inside says, "Hapy Brthdya!"

Now, obviously, there is a story behind this. One of the years that we were living at Nicholas', I decided I was going to do something nice by making my sister a "Happy Birthday" banner. I had kept it a secret until the day of, and then Mum helped me hang it up. The party was in full swing before some one finally noticed I had misspelled "Birthday" as "Brithday".

The adults started teasing me by wishing my sister a "Happy Brithday". I was embarrassed at first, but laughed along with everyone. Needless to say, I've remember how to correctly spell 'birthday' since.

Cam didn't think it was so funny, though. She ended up getting upset, and going to hide in our room. She only let her godmother go in to talk to her. Said godmother relayed the message that I had apparently ruined her entire birthday.

Huh... so that's probably when it started.

Fast-forward to last year. My sister was trying to help me through my birthday because of how upset I was. Yes, I plan to get into that story, but, again, I'm trying to not tangent. She and Grandma had bought a plain, vanilla cake. Then, Cam proceeded to decorate it, and made sure to put "Happy Brithday".

"How do you like it?" she taunted.

I just laughed. I honestly can't believe she's still holding the grudge against me for this long about a spelling error. The card was supposed to make reference to that, but I decided against purposefully antagonizing her. I think I'll save it for either Mum's or Grandma's birthday.

I can go on and on about the different shenanigans the pair of us has gotten into. I think I'm going to wrap this up with our trip to Canada's Wonderland about two years ago.

There's a ride there called *Wild Beast*. It's an old, wooden roller coaster. I like fast rides. I don't mind roller coasters, so long as there are not any high sudden drops. I detest the feeling of suddenly falling.

Let's just say suddenly falling triggers my anxiety in all the wrong ways.

Still, if it is not that steep on an incline, and not from very high, I may get myself to go onto the ride.

It was winding down that day, and Cam had her eyes set on *Wild Beast*. Neither of us had ever been on it before. From the spot where you get in line, a good majority of the coaster is out of view thanks to large trees. From what I could see, it was something that was just on the boarder of "not so bad" and "please, Heaven, no".

"Come on, there's no deep drops," she insisted.

I felt sick from what I could see, but her pleading tone roped me in. Once we were in line we got to see more and more of the coaster. Again, it did not look so bad, so my panic lessen. Enough that I let the brat also convince me to ride in the front row with her.

The train goes around to the raising platform. I already knew there were higher parts of the coaster, so I was not that worried. I figured the hill would turn into a small drop to add some speed, and then go through the rest. There were no loops, so I could handle it. At least that's what I was telling myself.

Almost to the top, we finally clear the treeline and can see the entire coaster. Include the single large drop on the other side of the hill we were currently going up.

"Holy shit," I squeak. "Are you FUCKING kidding me?!"

I look at Cam with my eyes the size of saucers. She is looking back at me pitifully, "I'm so sorry. I didn't know."

The car shudders to a slow crawl as we cross over the peak. I push my head fully against the back rest. I get a glimpse of the fall, and out tumbles, "You Bi..."

But then my mouth clamps shut because we're falling. I'm not sure if I was calling my sister, or fate, a bitch, but it was Cam's running joke for the rest of the day.

And, hilariously enough, after that initial drop, it was actually a fun coaster. So, at Cam's insistence, I got my ass back on it for a second ride. That hill was still Hell.

Honestly, I love that I have a sister. I love even more that I have Camilla as my sister. It doesn't matter how much she get's on my nerves, she's my best friend, and I dearly love her.

The Hail Mary Pass

I saw Nick Shepard Tuesday night. He was my first boyfriend, but we've been split for 6 or 7 years now. For the last year-ish, however, he's been hanging around. There's a long story to that, I don't feel like going through that spiel right now.

Nick was in St. Thomas and wanted to visit. Right now, there seems to be a game between us. He knows I want to push him out of my life. I've tried to do so repeatedly. At the same time, he is the only one that regularly talks to me. My family can leave me to my own devices for weeks at a time. When my mum does text me, it's just to check in that I'm still alive. I suppose that should be a comfort, but it doesn't exactly give me warm fuzzies either.

Nick texts me at 3:45 PM on Tuesday about a movie coming out. The texting lead to an unofficial request to visit, and I stupidly allowed it. He came over and stayed the night. I know he visits for the sake of sex. He is constantly telling me otherwise, but every single visit has resulted in it. I have a very hard time saying no. I know it's wrong, and without contraceptive, it's dangerous. Still, it's nice to be desired. Even if all he wants is a warm body since his latest ex left him.

I do try to detour him at times. Yet, as tired at he was after watching a 2-hour movie, he was magically energetic when I decided to go to bed. The game became more apparent when I told him I wanted to cut back. I told him I wanted to try and stop our visits all together. It's not the first time, but it doesn't really phase him anymore. Though I'm loathed to admit, we did commit the naked tango. He tries to be creative, with my prompting, but since it was his pushing that resulted in the coupling, it was one of those basic nights. Don't get me wrong. He never leaves me unsatisfied. Still, I've let these visits go on for too long. It's a relief when he leaves for work at 5 am.

Of course, then I feel drained afterwards. Self-hate bits

and claws at my self-esteem for letting things go too far again. I know I need to be stronger. If it wasn't for my appointments, I probably would have spent the day in my bed, and hoped my natural scent would eventually overpower the smell of shame and his cologne.

Certainly not a good mindset to start any day. It only added to my stress that Wednesday morning.

There was a sense of dread in my belly. It was the last day to withdraw from a class without being penalized; something I sorely needed to do because I have had horrible attendance this semester. Were I to stick with the classes that I was most behind in, and failed them, I would not be able to continue in the program.

The problem is, to drop even one course would make me a part-time student. As a part-time student, I lose my bus pass privilege, and my OSAP assistance. Without the latter, I would not be able to afford my rent, and the former means I could not get far to job search. I would have had to hope the couple of stores down the street from me were hiring.

I hate interviews. I hate how you must pretend you're truly interested in this base-level job. Meanwhile, you know and the employer knows that you only want the job to make ends meet. I've yet to meet anyone that's enthusiastic about getting a job as a cashier.

I had fucked up - big time. I missed so many classes. The thing is, I want to be there, be around kind and like-minded people. I want to better my skill set in Fine Arts. But, a lot of times, I just can't. I have no reason, aside from pure laziness. I feel like being clinically depressed is just an excuse. I know the truth is that I don't want to leave the security of my blankets, or the comfort snuggling with my cats bring. It's a battle because I know I must force myself to actually get out of bed, and fix my life. I'm the only one that can, after all.

I woke up Wednesday with the sense that I had waited too long to reach out for help. I should have gone to a counsellor the moment I realized I was falling back into my old routine. The same self-destructive path where I have one bad day, and I let it run me down into the heart of the kiln once more. You can't hold a job if you miss too many days, so you quit. That's how I ended up without a job for a year.

You can't attend school and expect to pass if your absent as often as you are present. I had started in September with the thought that I was going to break this cycle of letting doubt and insecurity sabotage me. By October, I knew better, but I kept it to myself until I was at a breaking point.

The thing is, the nurses and the counsellor can only help me so long as I'm a student at Fanshawe. With how I felt on Wednesday morning, I could count the days until the end of term in December. The only reason I bothered with my two appointments that day is because I would be charged $50 for not calling to cancel within 24 hours. I suppose that's one way to discourage no-shows.

I was back at the Clinic to go over a diet and exercise plan with a Nurse named Joy. Turns out, she's the one that attempted to draw my blood the first time I visited. Thing about mental health, they first have to do a crap tone of blood work to ensure it's not biological like thyroid or hormones. My lack of family doctor means I have to redo said bloodwork with every new clinic I visit.

Joy had completely missed the vein when she had done it. I don't hold it against her. Sticking someone with a needle was one of the things that turned me away from the RPN course.

Granted, I had not really wanted to be a Registered Practical Nurse. I wanted to make my mother proud. It was the one job option I told her about that didn't get nit-picked and ripped apart. Mum is very protective. She doesn't want me to fail, even to the point she holds me back from things that I could be successful at because, to her, the risk of failure is too high.

I can't say word for word what Joy and I talked about. I

know there were a few minutes there about some diet and exercise ideas. Things that I had heard plenty of times before. It was just another person putting me on the spot for the fact I eat and drink what I want, when I want, with no consideration of nutrition or the fact that diabetes does run on my family.

    Okay, that's not entirely true. There's always this nagging voice in my head about drinking pop or eating too much processed food. Every time I go to the grocery store, I try to buy items with the intention of healthy eating. Needless to say, the junk foods get eaten faster. Mostly because they don't require preparation to eat. I love the taste of a fresh, ripe mango, but skinning and chopping it is tedious. I have a juicy steak in my freezer, and some uncooked broccoli and asparagus in my fridge. It's nothing to steam the vegetables and grill the beef. Add a glass of strawberry milk, and some blueberries for dessert, and there you go. One healthy meal. The problem is, not even hunger motivates me enough to make it. I'm sure the asparagus has gone bad by now. It's been a couple days since I've looked inside my fridge.

    Just another way I'm letting laziness ruin my life.

    The rest of my conversation with Joy stepped a little into my worries about school. We tried to stay on topic, but the meeting ended up taking an hour. I had cried at least twice during the conversation. She did suggest I look into an alternative course. Fine Art Foundation had been an insecure choice, with no plans for the future once I completed it. If I completed it, that is. To be completely honest, I was just trying to do something with my life before I ended up homeless.

    By the time I had left that office, I had made up my mind to drop down to a part-time student. At least juggling a handful of classes gave me a chance to pass them, and then I might have a chance at starting a different course in January. I would probably need a job, too. One within walking distance, seeing as I wouldn't have use of my bus pass anymore. It felt hopeless, because there were too many "what if's." At least, it was a plan.

An hour and a half later, I headed for my second meeting with my new counsellor, Linda. She's a sweet soul. I can tell she genuinely wants to help people. I felt bad when, only a few minutes into our meeting, I start crying. I told her exactly what I had been thinking about school-wise. She stepped out a moment to ask if there was anything that could be done to help. The unfortunate fact I was not fully registered in accessibility – which is meant for people with various disorders, including crippling mental health – meant there was no way to leave a course without losing full-time status.

Basically, she confirmed what I had been worrying about all morning. That when my minor tearing up turned into bawling. By that point, my memory gets foggy. I can tell you that at one point I had growled out, "What's the point?" In my mind, I was going to fail school and likely end up facing homelessness again. I did, however, mention what Joy had said about finding a different class, but I back tracked just as fast.

"That won't work. Why would OSAP give me money towards a different class if I can't even finish my current one?"

Linda had gained a thoughtful look about her. She excused herself again, saying she had two more questions for the Academic Counsellor. I don't know what she went to ask. I know I was trying to calm myself down so I wasn't upsetting her. There was only so much she could do to help me. It's not fair to have one of my crying, hopeless fits in front of her when she was doing all she could.

Then, in the blink of an eye, Linda returned with another woman. Her name was Anita, and she rushed in with a quick introduction. She plunked herself down at Linda's desk where my school information was still open. Linda and I had been trying to find to see just how far behind I was before she had gone to speak with Anita... she said it might not be as bad as I thought.

Anita tried to determine which classes I was better

dropping, but I stepped in and told her exactly which three I had little chance of recovering. She wrote down the codes of each, and asked if I knew where a certain room was. I didn't. Neither did Linda. It *is* a fairly large school.

Anita said she'd take me, then quickly ushered me out the door. I looked back to Linda with confusion. She gave me a reassuring look, though she appeared to be about as flustered as I was by this sudden action. I raced after Anita. I wasn't sure what was going on. It sounded like she was going to help me with an academic plan. Which included removing the three classes from this semester, and doing them in fall of next year. The problem was, the deadline was the 16th at 4 pm. When she had come into Linda's office, it had already been 3:50-ish.

"Don't worry. It's going to be okay. We got this," she reassured me.

I didn't want to correct her in saying that doing this was going to make me a part-time student. I decided to just follow her lead. It sounded like she had an answer, after all.

I will say this, though: fuck she moves fast! For someone of my size, I'm a rather fast walker. This Anita, however, was doing a light speed walk, and I practically had to jog to keep up.

We made it to the other office with 5 minutes remaining. She asked the receptionist if Tina was still in. For the first time since meeting this woman, she seemed unsure if this was going to work. As it turned out, this mysterious Tina lady *was* still available, but she just had another person with her at the moment.

While we waited, Anita and I finished up some paperwork she had been working on during our trek. I think it was to officially have me sign up through Accessibility. I'm not entirely sure, though. At first, she had me sit down and was trying to instruct me what to say to Tina. I must have looked like a pitiful mess as I struggled to repeat the instructions. I was terrified that if this was going to fix things, I could not be the one to do it. Not on my own. I would fuck it up for sure. Mercifully, Anita stayed.

Tina turned out to be a rather nice lady as well. She and Anita joked about how crazy these deadline days always are. In no time at all, Anita was having Tina sign some papers, and I was freed from the three courses I was certain I was going to fail this semester.

I did get nervous though, and asked, "Is this going to make me a part-time student?"

"Oh, no!" Anita cheerfully answered. "Because you're registered with us, as long as you still have at least 40% of your course load, you're a full-time student as far as OSAP is concerned. See, I told you it's going to be okay. We've got this."

I was in complete shock. I said as much as we walked back to the counselling offices.

Anita joked, "This is what they call a Hail Mary pass in football."

I agreed, and even dared to smile. I silently praised God for his timing, and apologized for forgetting that He always has a plan. There was a reason I was to see both Joy and Linda that day. The suggestion of one, led to questions from another, which led to this whirlwind woman coming in and saving the day. Apparently, Anita is my new Academic/Accessibility Counsellor. I have an appointment with her next Tuesday at 4PM.

I still have to catch up in the remaining three classes, but I have enough confidence that I can do it. I know, in truth, it's not going to be easy, but it's a start. It's a plan. For the first time since October, I have hope again that I can, and will, complete this course. I won't be a college drop out for a second time.

What comes after school, though, well, now that my one-year course is being stretched into two, I have time to consider my options without panic. A lot can happen in that amount of time. Maybe I'll even finish my novel. I have plenty of time to write now.

It's amazing what a little bit of hope can do.

I have a new favourite song for the moment. *"(It's Gonna Be) Okay"* by the Piano Guys. I started listening to it a couple of days ago. There's just something reassuring hearing someone tell me (unintentionally) through music that:

No matter what you've been through, here you are. No matter if you think you're falling apart. It's gonna be okay.

The Black Sheep

It was a couple weeks after my sister's birthday that Mum called me. She sounded excited.

"So, you know how your birthday is the 19th. And its also Father's Day..."

Yes, the lovely side effect of being born in late June. Some years, I have to share my birthday with Father's Day. 2016 was one of those years.

"I found out that (some musician. I didn't care to remember) is playing at Caesar's Windsor. Do you want to go?"

My heart sunk. Mum knows I hate concerts. I didn't even know the artist to know if I could put up with loud music for a couple hours. I was sure it wouldn't be an artist I would enjoy at normal volumes. Mum and I have very different tastes in music, save for a few artists such as Bryan Adams, and Queen.

Further more, what about our over night trip? Was she honestly backing out on our plan because of some concert?

Turns out, yes. Yes, she was.

Still, a small hope within me tried to give her the benefit of the doubt.

"Well, I could stay in the hotel room while you went..." I tentatively offered.

"We're not staying overnight. I have to work in the morning."

"I thought you took the 20th off."

Mum immediately lost her cheery tone, "I thought you wanted to get your cat fixed for your birthday?"

About a week before, my torbie, Aurora, had been in heat. It was already the third time this year, and she was driving me nuts. I knew I had to scrounge up money to have her spayed, but until then, she was yowling for hours on end. I had jokingly texted my mother and sister, asking both if they could help me get her fixed as a birthday gift. Just some light humour to feel better. Apparently, Mum had thought I was serious.

"It was a joke," I told her.

We were both quiet a moment, then Mum scoffed, "I knew you wouldn't want to go. Your sister told me I should ask, anyway."

I cut in, "Well, you and I can do something else a different weekend."

Mum huffed again, "I'm already going with Grandma the weekend before to see Dolly Parton. I don't want to take too many weekends off."

By then, I was quiet, because I didn't trust my voice. I would have either started bawling, or had a few choice words. My mother had gone back on her word. I was not important enough to take an extra weekend off. I, apparently, wasn't even important enough to miss a concert for.

"We'll just go for Chinese buffet, alright?" she pressed.

"Fine." I hissed. I wanted that one word to tell her exactly how upset I was without saying so.

The call ended, and I spent the next hour crying. I got angry. Cam had to talk me down, and she and I decided that we would make my birthday special. We planned going to the YMCA with Tony and Kevin. I asked her to also ask Grandma if I could have a BBQ for the group of us at her house. I would buy the burgers, and we would stay in the backyard, out of Grandma's way.

Of course, it didn't play that way at all. Grandma eventually called me to day that she didn't want people over because it was Father's Day, and she was going to make a large dinner. Both Kevin and Tony had to cancel, because they already had plans with their fathers. As the day drew closer, I kept trying to figure out a way to salvage it. People were starting to get frustrated with me.

"Why does it *have* to be the 19th?"

"Because it's my 25th birthday. That's a big number." Honestly, that was the worst excuse I could have come up with. Everyone knew that's all it was.

How could I tell them, and make them understand, that after Mum chose a concert over me...

After Grandma chose a dinner over me...

After my sister decided I wasn't worth celebrating her birthday with, if it meant she got better treatment from everyone else...

After being left to wonder if the people I considered friends were even my friends at all...

I needed to feel like the day I came into existence actually meant something to someone else. To me, it meant that people gave a shit. That maybe, I am loved, and not just an obligation because I'm related.

But, one after another, no one had time for me. Not the 19th, anyway. Eventually, my sister opted we go fishing. Of course, we ended up relying on her boyfriend for a ride, and he didn't feel like going out until noon when we had planned for earlier. I give my sister credit for trying. She's the only one that did.

We got back from fishing mid afternoon. It gave us two hour before Mum came to pick up Cam and go to her precious concert. Since, you know, my sister does love concerts, and Mum wasn't going by herself. Grandma had most of her feast cooked and asked me to call Mum to see if she was coming over to eat before going.

Grudgingly, I did.

"We'll see. I still have a lot of stuff to get done around here."

She showed up five minutes before they had to leave.

My sister got two hours in between Mum working and running errands. I got five minutes, and she had had the whole day off. Long enough to hand me a card, and one of those over inflated balloons that are attached to a plastic straw. I took it in stride, and laughed when she went to hand me the balloon, and it came off it's stick. Then, she was going on about how excited she was about this concert. In the blink of an eye, she and Cam were gone for the hour drive to Windsor.

I sat quietly with Grandma working away in the kitchen, until my Uncle John and Aunt Sandra came over with the kids like they do every Sunday. They wished me happy birthday, and I got another card, but the rest played out like any other Sunday. We played cards. We ate. The kids had the TV going while they played their games.

I can't say my attitude about the situation didn't get through to my mother. Her apology was sending me camping at CM Wilson's conservation for two nights, at the end of the following week. It ended up being quiet, and had great fishing. Just what I needed to recharge.

Mum didn't camp with me, either. She did come out in time to enjoy the campfire each night, to visit and cook chicken pot pies. I invited my sister to join me the second night so I wasn't spending the whole time by myself. Thanks to an oversight in the pricing, I even arranged it that I could spend a third night.

I did have fun with my sister during the day, but apparently my laid back camper approach wasn't exciting enough for her. She ended up inviting her boyfriend out, even though I had told her not to when I initially invited her to join me. I knew he would get whinny about something, which would piss her off and make her difficult to deal with.

Sure enough, he dragged down the mood. I decided to take my rod out to go back fishing, and the two of them came with. This lead to him being pissed off because he wasn't catching the biggest fish. Which didn't matter, because we were throwing them back, anyway.

I did my best to ignore them. I didn't feel like placating my sister when her boyfriend got under her skin. Especially since this trip was meant for me.

I tried not to let on, but after the ordeal between mine and Cam's birthdays, I was keeping an emotional distance from Mum and Cam. It was harder to do with Mum. When she took me apartment hunting in London, we had had a great day, and she had been saying for a week before that we could go to the Comber fair. Except, her cousin called about going out on the water in her husband's boat. Just Mum, though. There wasn't enough room for me.

"We can go to the Western Fair instead. There will be more to do, anyway."

Except we didn't go to Western. The day she had off to go was one of the days the fair was closed. Thankfully, she didn't try to tell me we were going to do something else instead. I know my place in the family. An inconvenience, and a failure. It had been that way for as long as I can remember, but only became openly so when I dropped out of Nursing School.

Mum used to call Cam every day that she was away in Barrie. I know, because I was still living with her then. I'm lucky to get a text even once a week, asking me what I'm up too. She never shows interest in my answer, though. The most we chatted was when I was giving her a play-by-play of the London Santa Clause Parade on November 12th.

Honestly, it's the worst feeling in the world. I feel like my Mum only truly gave me attention when I was doing well in school, and getting awards. Once that was all gone, she didn't seem to care anymore. I know she loves me, as a mother does. It shows whenever she feels the need to protect me. But she doesn't show interest in me, as an individual. She talks down to me, as if I didn't already worry about finding a job, or doing well in school. She shows no interest in my art. Even less interest in my writing.

There was once a time, any time I mentioned my writing, her response was "cool". After I left the call centre, and started to pursue my writing more intently and passionately, she would change the subject if I brought it up. I started mentioning it just to see if she was doing it on purpose, and, never fail, she had something else to talk about every time.

It's not like she isn't a reader. I was named after one of her favourite authors, after all. I think the part that hurts the most is, there was a time one of the residence at the nursing home had asked her to read his work. Seeing her with the pages in her hand, listening to her talk about how she wished he would hurry up and finish the next page with such excitement. I don't know a worse slap in the face than that.

There's no way for me to tell her, without her misunderstanding, and having a fit. She doesn't listen to me. Growing up, if I had something to say to her, I wrote it in letters, because it was the only way to get it out without her cutting me off, and dismissing me.

Maybe one day I'll succeed at finishing, and publishing my novel. Then, I'll publish this. As a sort of autobiography, and she'll know exactly how I feel. She'd probably say that none of it is true, or that I'm being too sensitive, or something else. She'll never admit that one of the biggest reasons I hurt inside is because she can't accept who I am. She loves me as her daughter, but not as Anita Burns.

Honestly, it makes it very hard for me to love and accept who I am when my own mother can't.

5 AM

It's the 19th of November. Once again, I am wide awake at 5 AM. I enjoy that hour between 5 and 6. Back in Chatham, the town is silent. Most people are in their beds, including the drunken assholes. People on over night shift are nearing the end stretch, and morning shifters are just starting to rise. Even living in the centre of town, all man-made things are quiet. Humanity is quiet.

You can hear yourself think. You don't have to be anywhere, and no one is expecting anything of you. In the summer, bird song alerts you to the coming dawn. During the summer solstice, you can even witness the first rays of light climbing over the horizon.

In the winter, it's so quiet, you swear you can hear the wind whispering stories. I especially love 5 AM after a night of heavy snow fall. There's an indescribable sensation when a snow storm is starting or ending. I dare say it feels like peace. The same peace I feel at 5 in the morning. So, the two combined becomes something different. Magical, really. No matter the season, there is this unappreciated beauty about the hour. It could also be an instinctive relief that the night is ending. I don't know for certain, but I know that no amount of words can justify it.

5 AM is different here in London, though. There are still plenty of people awake. It's still the calmest point in the day, but there are more noises. Cars driving by, and the nearby trains are starting to move again.

I think I'm home sick.

I had gone out for a walk down the street to the store. Cozy in my fuzzy onesie, with my fall sweater over top, I was greeted by the scent of wet leaves and earth. It had apparently rained last night. I wish I could have paused to really take in the smell. I find earthy tones comforting. There's this tickle of nostalgia, coupled with a sense of awe and belonging.

There are a lot of spots in Chatham that reconnect me to that feeling. The creek near my mother's house during the fall, is one such place. There's a moment in the year when the banks are full of ducks and geese, and the leaves are vibrant, but haven't fallen. I took a picture of it once. I hope to recreate it as a painting someday.

It's nice that London has plenty to do. Not everything is closed down by 10 PM. But I am missing the quiet, and the autumn scent. The only thing working in London's favour is that it rains a lot. There's a magic to rain, too.

Maybe the city is adding to my anxiety. I don't feel like I can rest; not fully, anyway. I wish there was somewhere to go camping just so I can ground myself for a little while. All I have right now is 5 am, and rain.

The Step-Father

Holy Snow Miser, Batman!

Yes, I am very proud of that double reference.

In all seriousness, though, it's snowing! I don't mean the same light brushing that hardly covers the grass, like in Chatham. I knew coming up here that London would get more precipitation than Chatham. I remembered as much when the fall rain had started. I should have realized that the first snow fall in London was going to be exactly that. My weather app says it's going to carry on well into tomorrow. I hope it does. It will be Sunday, and I don't have to be anywhere. I can curl up with my blinds open, watching it all come down from the comfort of home.

I've already stood outside in it. I'm very grateful my new place has a balcony for moments like this. The sensation was there. That euphoric feeling of peace. Add in the sight of Christmas lights hanging on the balconies...

It's magic. Plain and simple.

I ended up watching *The Muppets Christmas Carol* as a means to make the feeling last longer. I should have plugged my Christmas tree in too. Except I was more concerned with chasing Cleo out of it.

My mind started wandering again. It does that a lot. I thought about tobogganing down the hill that was in our backyard when we had moved in with my temporary step-father, Nicholas. It made me think about him, and how I used to hate him. Honestly, what I hated was how he treated my mother. Unlike my biological father, he never laid a hand on her. But he was an intimidating man, and was prone to punching holes in the walls when he was angry. The master bedroom door had a dent for years where Mum had angrily tried to close the door on him during a fight, and he had slammed it open with the heel of his wrist.

He certainly did not make growing up easy. When it came to my sister and I, he was heavy handed in his punishments. Meanwhile, his sons were hardly ever punished. Of course, now that I think about it, he only had his two boys every other weekend, but me and Cam were under his full-time care. Perhaps that is one of the reasons. That, and, I wasn't exactly the best-behaved child, either.

For example, I was the one that led my sister, and the younger of his sons off to a construction site to play on the parked bulldozer. We were supposed to be at the park at the centre of the complex Mum, Cam, and I lived in after she had left Richard.

I don't know where Mum or Nicholas were at during all this. I know it was not uncommon for Cam and I to be sent to the park without Mum. The mid-90s was a lot more lenient on child supervision. It helped that you could almost see the park from the front window of our complex. Not far for scared little legs to run home, if need be. Plus, we had a lot of neighbours that had kids of their own. So, there were a lot of eyes on the park from sun up to sun down.

I don't think the neighbours knew who James was. He was the older of Nicholas' boys, though he still three months younger than myself. A fact that I would lord over him, any chance I got. I told you I was a little shit.

The worst part about me leading the two to our secret playground was that Cody, a boy who had to be about four or five years old at the time, was asthmatic. Plus, whatever age Cody was, my sister was a year younger. I could have very well lead a three year old off to a construction sight, near a major road. Thankfully, all of us ended up being fine.

In the end, it wasn't any of these factors that led to us being caught. It wasn't James tattling, or Cody's asthma, or even the neighbours seeing us (or rather, not seeing us). Cam had needed to run home for the toilet. The distance, combined with a young, tiny bladder led to her peeing her pants. Mum easily got it out of Cam that we weren't a short jaunt away at the park. Boy, was there Hell to pay.

Like I said, it's not as if we didn't deserve the punishments we got. It made me realize that, despite all his faults, Nicholas did do a better job at being our father than our actual sperm-donor (the fucking asshole). Granted, that was not a high bar to jump to begin with.

He was the one that taught me how to properly swing an axe when chopping wood. It's because of him I'm not squeamish around open wounds. I mean, he was a hunter, so it was not uncommon for him to have a carcase on the table. I remember one time I was helping him clean snapping turtle meat. He showed me how, even skinned and chopped into little pieces, the nerves could still be stimulated. Mum had come home while I had the foot in my hand.

I ran up to her, "Mom, watch this!" Then I proceeded to pull a nerve which caused the entire foot to bend its toes. Like a hand grasping for a baseball, and then letting go. I brought up this memory to her once, and she still shudders.

Nicholas even took us places. I don't know what trip was his idea and which was Mum's, but he never made excuses to sit out. He rode rides with us. He let us take turns learning to park his car. He encouraged me to fight back against bullies. He pushed me to not be afraid of horror movies- Though, admittedly, I still am. He worked to turn his little, single-level, two-bedroom home into three floors with more rooms for us four kids.

He was an aggressive asshole, but he was also a father figure.

Funny that the snow made me think of him. I don't know if this is just something I do, or if it's a depression/anxiety trait. Sometimes the slightest things, something as small as a snowflake, triggers a trip down memory lane- good and bad. If I'm completely honest, it get's exhausting fast.

A Sceptical Prophecy

It's 3 am on November 22nd. I'm supposed to be sleeping so that I am rested for class tomorrow, except my body wouldn't let me sleep past 2:30 am. Apparently, I want to be awake at night. Probably the fact it's quiet and way less stressful. This backwards sleep caused me to miss my 2D and 3D media class yesterday. I'm worried that I may end up continuing the pattern, and miss my classes still.

Honestly, sleeping for 14 hours is the dumbest reason to fail school.

A phone call from Mum today had taken a lot out of me too.

"The person that diagnosed you. Was it an actual doctor?"

"Yes. I even have her card," and then I started to read the doctor's accomplishments on the card. The first one clearly printed says 'MD'.

"Where did you meet her at?" Mum continues to press.

I already knew she was going to come out with something to piss me off, but I answer anyway. "She works through the school clinic."

"Well, I've just been sitting here thinking about it...And this woman is telling you that your depressed. So, lets cut back on classes so that you're at home alone more..."

I had cut her off by then. Figures my mother would stew on different thought trains to attempt to discredit someone trying to help me, instead of accepting that I actually do have mental health concerns. Cam is already diagnosed and medicated for being bi-polar. If I have mental health issues too, then it looks bad on Mum's parenting.

That one line had me reeling. Not only was she implying the doctor was a pill pushing quack, but I was just being impressionable, and don't know my own mind.

I stopped the spiel, and very clearly made my point (seething all the while), "It was my choice. I have been getting stressed, and I'm falling behind on my classes. This way, I stand a chance at getting good marks."

She was quiet for only a heartbeat, "But it's going to take you twice as long."

"Then it takes me twice as long," I quip. "It's not like I'm doing anything else with my life."

Pause. "Yeah, but it's going to cost twice as much."

"Then it costs me twice as much. I would rather get better marks..." what I meant by that is that I'd like to actually pass. "And use it to get into whatever program I want. Besides, a lot can change in two years. I might decide to continue, or I might go into Advance Film Making. They have that here. It's like the course I was trying to get into the Vancouver Film School for."

There wasn't much else to our conversation. I'm sure Mum will have more to say later. The thing is, mentioning VFS triggered another memory. The only reason it had been a goal was because of some psychic.

I don't much believe in psychics. I wonder, plenty, if there is a supernatural ability to tell the future in us. I know for a fact I have had dreams of moments that did not make sense at the time, but later turned out to be a glimpse of something I see sometime later. I'm not sure if it's my imagination, or if I'm using a mixed up, not-all-there dream as an excuse for my deja vu. I'm sure there's at least a hundred logical, and less supernatural reasons for the sensation, but it's something I can't deny experiencing more than once.

I had always wanted to see a 'genuine' psychic, to find out if there was any truth to it. Mum decided that, for my 22nd birthday, we would see one that she and Heather had seen when they were younger. Mum swore by this woman. Which is saying something, because my Mum is pretty quick to call out a liar. Aunt Heather seemed a little baffled. Like she wanted to be sceptical, but could not ignore there had been something causing her pause.

Here's the kicker. At that point in time, even Mum could see I was sinking further into depression. It's why she had decided on a psychic that year.

"You just need some hope."

We pull into this woman's drive, and I put on a stone face right away. I do know one thing these 'mystical' people have in common; they're observant. They have to be in order to bullshit someone into believing their future is being told. I wanted to remain as plain as possible, and see what she would tell me.

When I handed her my keys, 'to read my energy', she jumped. She slyly grinned, "My, you have a very strong soul."

I could not help smirking a little. I have to give the woman credit for her theatrics. She was going to make the next hour entertaining, if nothing else.

She continued, "It's an old soul. You have lived hundreds of lives before this one. You have been male as many times as you have been female. In some lives you were rich, and others you were poor. In every life you were a rebel of some form. Many times, you were the leader. There were also many times you were in chains. It's why you don't like bracelets. They make you feel constricted."

I remember that line because I had to admit to myself, the bracelet bit was true. Not the part about it relating to memories about times I was in chains, but that they make me feel constricted. I use my hands and arms a lot (drawing, sculpting, fidgeting, etc.), so I don't like them being inhibited.

I also don't like necklaces or tight collars either. I'm hyper aware of something against my neck, and it causes me to itch and feel like I'm chocking. I've gotten better with necklaces, and wear them when I feel like bedazzling myself, but, for the most part, I don't. Same goes for earrings, or just make-up in general. Those, however, I just find as tedious annoyances.

The psychic woman did have to make a point about the fact I wasn't wearing a necklace that day. After she mentioned the bracelet and chains bit, she got this look of concern. Her hand gently touched her throat, and she said with a small quiver, "You have a sensitive neck. You were, well, you've been beheaded many times." I think she had given a reason how my previous life beheading related to current neck sensitivity, but I can't remember. I was definitely amused, though.

"You're a writer."

That one had taken me off guard. In fact, it took me a few months later before I realized she could have seen the notebook in my back pack while I reached in to get my keys at the start.

Like I said; observant.

I confirmed it, a little taken back.

"You write fantasy." The pair of Digimon key chains could have easily given away that I was into make-believe things.

"They're real, though. You write about battles that are based on real fights that you have been apart of. You have worn the armour your character wears."

At the time, my character wore a breast plate over an outfit similar to Shang dynasty It looked a lot like the armour worn in Disney's *Mulan* (one of my favourite movies). I went through a phase where I was really into Chinese art, and Taoism. I had learned a couple phrases, as well, but the only things I remember now is how to say "hello", "I love you", and "son of a bitch." I would still like to go, and learn more about the culture and history from the actual people some day.

Also, my character, Autumn, has since gained a more Western-style outfit as my artistic interests have changed to Romanesque architecture and design. That was a conscious choice, but nice try psychic lady.

She also correctly guessed that it was about a hierarchy. I, always one to love talking about my book, smiled and told her it was about a kingdom of angel-like creatures. I didn't get farther than that because I remembered I was supposed to remain stoic, and not give away too much.

She seemed satisfied with pulling that bit of information out of me, because (after about 20 minutes of talking about these supposed past lives) she finally got into talking about the future.

"Have you ever considered getting into the justice system? I can see you as a judge or lawyer or an officer..."

"No," I laughed.

At the time, I didn't know where I was going or what I was doing with my life. I just knew I didn't want to stay at the call centre forever. Mum had been pushing the idea of boarder security, along side dietary aid, and food inspector. It always came down to "I was talking to so-and-so, and they said it's only a year of schooling, and you'd be making good money."

I think that's part of the reason Mum doesn't like the idea of me being in school twice as long as originally intended. Especially on a course that doesn't have a guarantee job market. Whenever I brought up plans for school, or job desires, they were always scrutinized into her main three categories; length of schooling, job availability, and money.

My categories are: is it challenging enough without making me over anxious? What is the pay off should I succeed? Will I enjoy it?

I don't worry about money, because any full-time job (even one on minimum wage) is enough to get me by, and still be able to save a large wad for retirement and trips.

Mum does not like that I would be in school until I am 31. I think she thinks I expect her to help throughout it too. Honestly, I appreciate that she brings me groceries from time to time, but she doesn't have to do it. Mothers will be mothers, I suppose. I just want to be able to enjoy whatever it is I'm stuck doing for the rest of my life.

When the psychic had mentioned cop, I had instantly thought of Mum, and her push for boarder security. Thus, I had laughed while saying 'no'.

She thought for a moment, and then said, "Well, you do have a second path before you. This one will be long and difficult. I see you as a famous director. You'll move West, and you will create masterpieces as great as Steven Spielberg, and James Cameron. You're name will be on TV screens across the country. But first, you will write. I see you finishing 3 to 6 books, and they will launch you into the film industry. Until they are done, though, I see you struggling. You will jump from job to job just to make ends meet."

I had not really heeded the warning. I was in a fairly well-paying job. I was smart, and confident, and believed that I had already jumped from job to job enough to count. I still carried teenaged arrogance, and thought I knew better.

I have always loved movies. I'm constantly watching the behind the scenes of my favourites to get into the head of the creators. The amount of time, effort, and teamwork that goes into these productions... I'm awe struck every time. Sometimes they can take several years, for something we enjoy over the course of 3 hours, at most.

I loved the idea that I could make my ideas into a reality. I could be on a set, getting hands on in all the departments. Creating these grand stories meant to capture the imagination, and entertain people. The ability to pull at heart strings, make imaginary people real, and all while working along side just as enthusiastic people.

Doing a little research after my visit to the psychic, I learned that if you wanted to be somebody in the Canadian film industry, Vancouver was the city to be. Toronto is a very close second, but it was too close to home for my wander-lust.

Vancouver was a place I had never been, settled between mountains on one side, and the ocean on the other. I had not really considered commuting, but I should have since I know living in Vancouver would drive me batty. I swear, London is already too urban for me.

I stayed at that call centre far longer than my mental health could handle. I scrimped and saved as much as I could. It would have been my entire paycheck if Mum wasn't demanding a third of it for room and board.

There was a time Mum was letting me live rent free for a while, but then she got pissed off at me over some fight or another that we had. I can't remember what is was about. I'm sure she does. She knew I was stuck either giving her the money, or paying more to rent my own place. I get she can't help it, but her and her damn control issues, I swear.

Needless to say, after two long years (worked a total of 25 months in that Hell hole), I had saved almost $13,000. A large sum of cash, but not even half of what I needed to go to the Vancouver Film School.

What happened was, I got tired of being an adult living under my mother's thumb. I spent $2,500 of my savings to pay first and last for my own place, and buy all my needed furniture and utensils. I'm sure it would have cost way more to start out, but my Aunt Heather is a thrift store ninja master.

Once I was free to live as I pleased, I decided the money earned was not worth the mental trauma that comes from working in a complaint call centre. I mean really, is it that hard to be considerate of the poor soul that has the misfortune of representing a product you are currently not happy with? I could go on and on, but let's sum it up to: I think I would prefer cleaning port-a-john's at a chili taco festival than work for another complaint centre.

Still, I took my savings, and I decided that I would give being a full-time writer a shot. I actually got really far too, until the money started to run out, and I panicked. Thus began the true hardship of my adult life.

    I don't know how much of what that 'psychic' had said would be true. Whenever I need a bit of hope though, I tell myself that I am the hero of my fantasy, and her words were my prophecy to let me know that the darkness will end. A clever little lie, but it get's me through the day. Like Mum had said, I just need a little hope.

Brushes

It's 4 am on the 24th of November. The last two days have been a whirlwind. I didn't make it to my painting class on Tuesday. I was awake, and wanted to go, but it felt dumb to go to class without at least one of the two projects I'm supposed to have done by now, completed. Almost as if I was insulting my teacher, and using my mental health as an excuse to not have them done.

So, after my appointment with Anita that day, I went to the classroom to work on one of the paintings. I had one, a self-portrait, that was nearly completed. It took me three hours, but it's finished. I'm also in love with my new brushes. I usually get the cheapest I can, and use them for as long as the bristles hold out. Which, when using dollar store acrylic paints, can be a while. A few weeks back, however, Mum tells me she has Michael's Craft Store coupons.

Michael's is a very dangerous store for me to walk into at any time. My budget hardly ever allows me use of such high-end items, and the store, I've been told, is among the more expensive of craft stores. I'm sorely tempted to buy and try what I can. My painting class has been very hard on my cheap brushes this year. Apparently, they can't handle actual acrylic. It's been a nightmare making sure they are clean, and, somehow, they're still stiff when I use them next.

Mum had asked if I needed anything for school from the store. I was hoping to convince her to let me use the coupon towards a new set of cheap brushes. I could not afford them at full price, but at 50% off, I could manage.

I, honestly, told her I needed new brushes. She knew I already had some, and asked about those ones. I got nervous. I thought that if I told her the truth, she would think I was not taking care of my brushes. I didn't want to be nagged at for something that was untrue. Nor did I feel like defending myself. So, I told her one of the problems I was having with them - the bristles are sticking in the painting - and played it off that it was getting me poorer marks in class. The truth is, we work in such large scale, you can hardly tell there are bristles in the painting until you look at it up close.

Mum did not give me the coupon, though. Instead, Aunt Heather printed us some 40% off coupons, and then Mum took me to Michael's to buy me the good brushes.

Yeah, that surprised the heck out of me.

I decided to only ask for four. Then I would have the basics: a fan, a half-inch square, and two detail brushes (one fine tip, the other square). We were only allowed one coupon per person, however. So, I resigned to a fan and a half-inch. Mum, however, decided we would just go back the next day and get the other two.

She did this a couple times, and she kept pushing about if I was sure these were all I needed. They were. I told her as much. But she would hold up another, and say, "Well, what about this one?"

My mother's stubbornness can be a headache, at times. Still, it helps since I don't generally ask when I need something. I eventually admitted to her that, no, I did not need the brush she was holding up, but I did want it. In the end, I ended up with 8 beautiful, professional grade brushes. I don't know if I thanked my mother enough times, but I know she waved it off every time I said it.

I had used them to finish my project yesterday. The way they glided with the paint, and easily twisted that I could make details my stiff old brushes could never have mustered... I was memorized. I have never been one to believe the saying, "an artist is only as good as their tools". For the first time in my life, I have the correct utensils in my hands, and I finally get the saying.

Seriously, I need to think of a way to properly thank my mother. Those 8 brushes were not cheap. Even with the coupons. Of course, now that I'm thinking about it, Mum never did go cheap when she got me art supplies for Christmas. She may not approve of me being a writer, but she seems to be supportive of my drawing and painting. Maybe I'm not a complete write-off to her.

Dig Deep

I don't know if this is a thing specific to me, or if it is a side effect of the mental health, but I tend to relive memories a lot. Many times these adventures are unwillingly set upon me. Nightmares of mistakes, moments of embarrassment, or just the haunting echo of cruel words. Last night, though, was one of few pleasant jumps.

I thought about another bout of mischief that James, Cody, Cam, and I had gotten into. Mischief that I had likely gotten us into.

It was sometime in early spring. The hill in our backyard was slick and muddy. It had to have been still new. I don't know for sure, but I do know that grass had not grown on it, yet.

You can imagine, the giant mound of unsettled dirt. Freshly melted snow making enormous puddles. Then, add in four outdoorsy children, who were told to stay off it. Needless to say, we didn't listen. It was one thing to mess around in the mud on the firm ground. The hill, though...

It was fun for the first couple minutes. We would sink down a little, and then pull our boots free with a *slurp*. We would laugh, and do it again. We had no worry about how we were going to explain the dirt coating on us, or the foot prints in the mud going up the hill. It was just fun.

Then James and I, being the older, bolder, and heavier of the four of us, had gone a little higher up the side of the hill. The loose earth shifted, and we got stuck nearly to our knees. It stopped being fun. We struggled, and wiggled thinking we could come loose like we had been doing. Our movement was only causing what little air-pocket we had around our feet to fill with mud. Which held us in place all the tighter.

For some reason, we thought dumping water from the plastic sled would get us loose. My best guess is that we thought it would wash the dirt away. All it did was cause the dirt to sink more while simultaneously eliminating the last of the air pockets. There was no getting out of it without digging. Except James and I were trapped in such a way that we could not bend to dig. We dare not sit, either, because we could have ended up stuck that way too.

Cody and Cam did what they could to help, but they could not come too close. I don't know if it was our yelling, or if one of the younger two had finally gone to get help, but it was Mum that came to the rescue. Except she could not get too close, either.

Eventually, she moved the plastic sled in between us, and had James and I get in, without our boots. Part of our punishment was that we had to dig them out ourselves before we could go inside, and get out of our muddy clothing.

Talk about learning earth science the hard way.

You know, this wasn't the only time I ended up with my shoes needing to be dug up. I just remembered the time I went with my scout group to Michigan to sleep in a submarine. Oh boy, that was a disaster.

I can't recall how young I was when I first joined Scouts Canada (originally Boy Scouts). I was young enough that I was part of the cubs group. I was young enough to believe that a "pack howl" was literally howling. It was also early enough from the switch between "Boy Scouts" and "Scouts Canada" that I was the first and only girl in St Joseph's Pack 17, and Troop 17 for a couple of years.

Being the only girl in a group of guys (including mostly male leaders) increased my competitive nature. It's like I had something to prove, all the time. There were plenty of times though that I didn't feel like putting up with the boys, and would go do my own thing. One of our stops during the Michigan trip was one such case.

We were at a beach, but the weather was chilly. Either late fall or early spring. There was no way we were going swimming, but there were sand dunes. Lots and lots of sand dunes. The boys went off to run up one side of the dunes, jump, and then slide down the other side. I, however, plunked myself at the bottom of one of the dunes, and started digging.

I don't know why it was so fun, but, in my youth, I was a digger. My running shoes were off, and a few feet away from me. I have no idea why I did what I did. The best I can recall, I thought I was keeping them safe. As you've likely guessed, I proceeded to bury my shoes in the hole. Then moved over a little, and started digging a new one.

You know, I can see why I was picked on as a kid. I had a very unique way of thinking, and doing things. I'm smirking now, because it's hilarious, and I am really questioning younger me's sanity. It took a long time before I got to live this one down. I can't believe I actually forgot about it for a while.

Fast forward a little, and it was time to go. Except, I no longer knew where I had buried my shoes. You would think I could tell because that was where the dirt was disturbed. Except, not even ten minutes prior, the boys had been by to do their jump and slide on the dune I was digging in. Thankfully, I was able to tell from my position compared to a nearby park the approximate area.

It took 17 people (scouts and leaders together), one and half hours, a reward bribe to motivate the boys to help, and six feet of digging, to finally find my damn shoes. It probably wouldn't have been so long, or dug as deep if we hadn't started at the top of the dune, but we were being thorough.

The two boys that found them ended up getting Michigan hot chocolate mugs, and bragging rights. There was even talk about nicknaming me "shoes". I think that was about the point I stopped being a digger. Unless you count the shallow digging needed to get to the good sculpting sand at a beach.

You know, I don't think I had an unhappy childhood. I may not have had a lot of friends, and was bullied in school, but I had my siblings to play with. My father wasn't a father, but I did get a step-dad that was okay. Mum did what she could to let us experience the world through trips, and such. I mean, how many kids had that opportunity? Even working as hard as she did, she still found time to watch a movie, work on a puzzle, or play board games.

I had plenty happen to me as a child, but I wasn't unhappy. Not truly. I had enough going for me to counter what was against me.

Maybe that's the root of it. I started heading into a depression when I lost the things that made me happy. I don't have a father. Mum had to work a lot to compensate for the missing party, and so I barely had my mother. The boys that were my brothers for 6 years weren't my brothers anymore. My sister and I grew to be as different as day and night. Our fun and games turned into mostly bickering and jealousy. That was on top of being bullied, and dealing with just the normal stresses of growing up. I had things. Plenty of inanimate objects to occupy myself with. But I didn't have people.

A counsellor once asked me if my greatest fear was being alone. At the time, I told her "no" because I was by myself a lot. It happened so much by then, I wasn't scared.

But I think I get it now. She was asking me if I was afraid of being alone in an emotional sense. Not having people regularly in my life. Was I afraid of loneliness?

Truthfully... Yes. I am. And it's a feeling that happens far too often. The question now is, how do I fix it?

Climbing Everest in the Buff

It's 7 am, November 25th. I'm not really sure what I want to do today, but I do know I'm supposed to do a 1/2 hour walk every day. I feel bad for Joy. I had an appointment with her on Wednesday. She's a nice enough individual, but trying to convince me to break my bad habits by simply telling me they are bad (which I already know), makes me bluntly honest about how unlikely it is to happen. Not because I don't want to go for a walk. Just because I don't have the motivation to do so.

"I can sit here and say, 'oh yeah, I'll definitely do it!', but I probably won't get far," I told her.

I know I frustrate a lot of people when I get this way. I'm not trying to be difficult. I am not entirely sure why I do it, but there was one person who seemed to understand it. The Chaplin that acted as a counsellor for me when I was in high school (on top of my actual counsellor).

She once pointed out, "You're just looking at all the honest options, good and bad, but I know you are listening to what I'm telling you."

That made sense to me. If I already know I'm going to act a certain way, why not see if they have a suggestion to counter it? My mother hates it. She's the only person I don't ask alternating questions with. It leaves me frustrated, but, at least then, we don't start to bicker. Joy doesn't know that about me, though.

She tried to help, regardless. I'm thankful to her for that. She told me about programs in the city that I didn't know existed. Hiking groups, for example. She pointed out some good walking and fishing trails nearby, as well. I should see where you can buy bait around here, and then head over. Maybe that is what I'll do today, if this rain will let up.

I also saw Anita, again. We met on Tuesday, after I was

supposed to go to class. I felt ashamed to admit I had not gone, again. After some talking, she helped me realized that I was not intimidated, but embarrassed to face my teachers when I'm so far behind. That does make sense. The first couple times I had missed class was because I was feeling overwhelmed, and needed a rest day. It's why I had missed Fridays the most because I was just that exhausted by the end of the week. After that, though, I didn't want to face my teachers without being caught up. It felt like anything else would be insulting them as professors. Perhaps it was a childish instinct to not want to be scolded for falling behind. Feels like it was both.

I like Anita. She has a wild, and cheery temperament. It's very hard to feel negative around her. Her favourite phrase seems to be, "You got this" or "We've got this". Honestly, the second makes me feel hopeful. The first, however, always makes me cry. I can say it to myself, plenty of times, but it just feels dull. When someone else looks me in the eyes, and says it, I cry. Thus far, every time.

After talking with Anita, she seems to believe the reason I cry is because I'm missing that support system. I don't talk to my friends enough to hear it from them. Most of my family doesn't say it. Either they think I already know, or, mostly in my mother's case, they think the exact opposite, and feel the need to nag and baby me. Really, all that does is piss me off, and make me feel worse. To think someone out there has listened to the crap I have gone through, and how I'm in a self-sabotage cycle, and, yet, they still believe in me. That "I've got this"... Well, I'm tearing up a little just writing this.

Maybe there is a large part of me that feels like I have to face the world alone. I try not to burden my loved ones so much that I don't think they know even half of what is going on in my head. The exception is my sister. As different as we are, we seem to have this bond that survives every one of our fights.

That may come off as a surprise, but I don't, nor have I ever, hated my sister. Our relationship is incredibly complicated because we are so different. We do get jealous of one another plenty, but I'm glad to have her in my life. I do love her, and I know she loves me.

She is the only one I trust enough to tell what I'm feeling to, but I'm wary to do so. She's betrayed my trust by telling Mum things I've said before. She is also prone to cut off from me in fits of anger, because she knows it'll really hurt me to just ignore me.

It's possible that this is why I am constantly looking for positive attention. At the end of the day, we all just want to be loved and accepted for who we are. When we don't get that, we react in so many different ways. I'm part of the group that grows to be ambitious. If you think about my biggest dreams, they all come down to the desire to be loved, supported, and even praised.

Write a novel that captures the imagination, and love of as many readers as I can.

Be financially successful enough that I can help, and spoil my loved ones.

Find my soul mate, and have a family.

Do some form of Missionary work (most likely helping save wildlife).

In the correct wording, that all sounds lovely, and maybe even selfless. Up front, when I see that I'm using good to get love and respect, it's all rather selfish. Guess I'm not as nice a person as I thought.

I might still be, to be honest. I do what I can for others, just because they might need help. It doesn't have to be some grand thing. Sometimes it's just politely holding the door open, or offering to help carry something heavy. Yet, most of the things I hope to do with my life, I have a hard time thinking of how to do them anonymously. It's like I need another person's gratitude, no matter how small and brief, to give me purpose.

It's possible that it's not quite it. Usually, when I think of helping someone, I'm actually concerned about making their lives easier or happier. Even for just a moment in time. Still, is there an underlining selfishness to each deed, this entire time?

You know this brings me to my last appointment this week. I had a last minute scheduling with Linda. During our meeting, she asked me if I'm letting the thoughts and feelings of others control me too much.

A 'trigger', she called it. I usually refer to those as my "twitches".

She is not the first person to tell me this, but I keep needing to be reminded. Loneliness can do terrible things to the mind. Home is less a safe haven, and more a prison. Yet, leaving it, you go out into a world that doesn't understand your way of thinking. That's the side effect of being an artist. You do things your own way, and it makes you an outsider. Then you get lonely, and doubt yourself. You can't really love yourself properly, so you do what you can in hopes that someone, somewhere will accept and love you. When they don't, you just doubt yourself more.

On and on the cycle goes.

There was once a time I believed in myself. I told myself the world didn't know what they were talking about. I was fantastic the way I was.

Then one day, either loneliness or doubt took that away. I don't know how to get it back for myself without help. To fit in, I would have to change, or, at least, come up with a clever disguise. Which negates the point of searching for someone to understand and accept you as you are. After a while, you're not sure anymore who you are, or if that person inside is even worthy of affection. What a toxic way to live.

The easy answer to all of this is to love yourself for who you are. I don't know how to do that, right now. Linda had told me, though, that I need to take notice of my triggers. When I start in on something that puts myself down, even if it's just worrying about someone else's happiness, I need to remind myself it's a trigger, and leave it alone.

She might as well have told me to climb Everest in the buff, and without any gear.

As daunting as it sounds, I do feel hopeful. So long as I continue in school, I'm not alone. A cynical side of me wants to say it's just their jobs. Thing is, their jobs are to help me succeed in school. Being nice, and understanding is who they are.

I had a counsellor once that you could tell it was just a job to her. As soon as the session started, she would get a bored look on her face. She hardly said a word. I met with her a total of five times, and felt no better. Our last meeting, she told me she would call me in the new year to see how I was doing. If she felt I was doing fine, she would close the case.

She had never called. For the longest time, it made me feel like I must have been exaggerating my feelings. Like I was just being a whinny, spoiled brat. That was about three years ago. This is the first time since then that I had sought out mental health assistance. Considering I had had a regular counsellor since elementary school, that is saying something. I was not even that hopeful that Linda could actually help me when I first met her. I figured I was going to be allowed to vent frustrations every couple of weeks, and then go back to working through it alone.

Now, I have four different people keeping tabs on me.

Dr Adams

The nurse, Joy

My academic counsellor, Anita

And my personal counsellor, Linda

How's this for doing what they can to help: When I met with Anita, she had asked me if I had had another appointment with Linda.

"Yes, but it's not until the 9th," I admit.

Anita hummed, "Ooh, that is kind of far from now. Here, let me e-mail Linda to see if she can squeeze you in sooner." So, she sent the e-mail, right there in front of me.

Linda called me the next day, asking if I was free for 2 pm.

It was the same thing with Joy, and Dr Adams. During my meeting with Joy, she had done a survey. While I was leaving the office, Dr Adams waved me goodbye, and then pulled Joy aside to talk. I didn't hear all of it, as I was supposed to leave, but I did hear, "Does she need..." as the opening line. Unless there was another she that I didn't know about, I assume they were reviewing my meeting for when I meet with Dr Adams on Monday.

It feels nice to have someone watching my back. My own personal A-team. Great, now I'm giggling about who is which character. Not sure about the other characters, but I think Anita would definitely be Murdock (he's my favourite character, by the way). I don't know if she would be flattered or insulted by the comparison.

I think that line was supposed to be considered a trigger.

Oh, and I did go to class on Wednesday. Maybe, just maybe, I've got this, after all.

Monsters, Screamers, and Creepers

It's 5 am on November 29th. I'm currently writing this with my sister playing on her Xbox (that she brought with her) on my couch. She's staying over until the 1st for something relating to her job. Some sort of training thing, from what I know.

Thus far, things have been good between us. We're not ready to kill each other, anyway. I think we'll be fine, though, since the two of us have our separate plans. We'll be spending enough time apart to not get on each other's nerves.

I had visited Chatham this past weekend. Mum had called me earlier in the week to say I should catch the train on Thursday, and then stay until she drives me home on Sunday. With the number of projects I have due, and knowing that being under my mother's roof for too long will bother me, I really did not want to spend my entire free time in Chatham. A weekend trip was one thing, but four days is another matter.

Speaking with Linda on Wednesday, she asked me if it was what I wanted. When I told her 'no' she suggested I should tell my mother that.

"And have her throw a fit?" I joked.

She told me to use an excuse then. I've never in my life heard someone encourage me to use the coward's route when facing a problem. An excuse, I could do, though. I try to be an honest person, simply because the truth comes out eventually. I can lie, however. I tell people I can't lie worth a damn, and there are plenty of grand lies or ones on the spot, that cause me to stumble and stutter. But I am a practised liar. It's a self-preservation instinct whenever I get too stressed.

The truth was that I needed to make an appointment to do work and safety lessons with our wood shop technician in order to complete my last sculpture project. I used that as my base to lie. I told Mum that we had to sign up for this lesson between the two days, Friday at 4 and Saturday at noon. 4 was when all the art classes were out for the day on Friday. Noon just seemed like a reasonable time for one to do such a class on a Saturday. I told her that I had already signed up the Friday one.

At first, Mum's reaction was to rush me to get on the Wednesday train, and then she would bring me home on Friday instead. That's why I added the bit about already being signed up. She said that maybe I should wait until her next weekend off, two weeks from now. I was disappointed. I wanted to see my home and family. I just thought 4 days was excessive.

It turned out that the lie had worked out for the better. Anita called me at 1 to ask if I could be at the school for a 2 o'clock meeting with my program coordinator, Gary. Turns out it was him and one of the full-time teachers for the Fine Art program, Marla.

I do like Marla. You can tell she wants her students to do well. She scares me, though. She has an air of authority that can be intimidating. The meeting was more to confirm that I can progress through as a full-time student under permanent disability.

I didn't like being under Gary's eye. He was scolding me about not going to my classes when they were making things easier for me. Add in Marla's authority beside me, it was Anita's presence that kept me from reacting with fight or flight. I did cry a little during the meeting while we were reviewing my marks. By that point, the unsettled feeling in my gut was just getting to be too much.

Thankfully, the meeting ended, and I was able to run off to the library to work on one of my projects. I had finished up by 5, and decided to text my mother pretending that I had just got out of the shop. She changed her plan, and told me I should take the next possible train to Chatham. It sounded like her idea, but, in the end, the set up was exactly what I had been aiming for.

The weekend had been nice. My mother is obsessed with the app, Pokemon Go. Any time we were not visiting my other family members was spent playing this game. I'm not a huge fan, but I do like to play it with my Mum. It's one of the few things we see eye to eye on, and let's me spend time with her. I got to spend hours just laughing about non-sense with her. I really enjoy those times.

We did meet a new friend while playing as well. Mum had apparently been teaming up with him for a few weeks now in taking over gyms, but the two of them had not met until Saturday morning. His name is Chris, and, apparently, he knew me.

I'm glad he remembered. I knew that I recognized him, some how, but I could not place where. Once he told me that he had been the monster in the cage, I remembered his black and white make-up. It looked like something akin to the guys from KISS. His scare spot was past the main dungeon, during the small maze into the third act. He also trained the other "monsters".

This was at Gregor's Crossing Haunted Dungeon, by the way. A home away from home for me during Halloween weekends back when I was in high school. This meeting with Chris sent me into another of my reliving memories when I tried to sleep that night.

I had tried various spots in the dungeon, myself. My first day, when I walked in to say I was a new volunteer, they put me in the Gallous. I had no idea what that was until they were strapping me into a harness, put a jacket over top to cover it, and then attached the back of the harness to a hanging post. I don't like the feeling of dropping. It pushes all the wrong buttons in me. Yet, there I was. My entire first day, the floor would be pulled out from under me, and I had to pretend I was hanging from my neck and not a harness under my jacket.

Mercifully, we got more volunteers, so I didn't have to be

the one hanging any more. I was the one pulling the floor loose. That got boring, so they put me on fog detail instead. When I got a little too excessive with the fog (our own people couldn't see very well), they moved me into the main dungeon.

That's the thing about Haunted Houses. Everyone has a certain way of doing things. It takes dozens of people to do various things. "Monsters", like Chris, were the ones that roar and scream in a visitor's face. "Screamers" are the pretend victims. They have to be able to scream loud enough for the people in the back to know to be ready.

When I was in the dungeon, I was put in a Screamer cage. That one involved pretending I was being disemboweled, and then the Dungeon Master would pretend to eat one of my organs. Whichever replica I kept hidden in my hand to the side. I usually grabbed the heart. It was the most distinctive one in the bucket vs a stomach or liver, and it made the dungeon master look like a sadistic creep.

Well, more of one, anyway.

It was all a sort of rubbery-plastic, by the way. No real blood or body parts were used. I still think he should have got some sausage links or the like, and pretended to pull out the intestines while the Screamer was "still alive". Then he could actually bite into it, verses just pretending. He probably would have gotten full fast, though.

You know, for a bloody coward, I'm pretty good at coming up with gruesome/creepy crap for fun. I tone it down a fair bit with my novel, but if I ever do make it into the film industry, I have a number of horror movies in mind. Comedy horror, though. I like audiences to have as much fun experiencing something as I do in making it.

I really miss the Haunted Dungeon. It was discontinued a long time ago. I miss the people. For a bunch of individuals that like scaring other people, we were all super nice, and all around friendly.

I miss getting to dress up in costume too. My final year,

they had found out that I did best as first scare. I would wait in a quiet corner, as silent as I could. Sometimes, I would turn "monster" on the first person in the line up. Mostly, I was a "creeper", which is a silent follower that touches someone's shoulder, or suddenly screams. Sometimes, I got really mean, and went for the people in the middle. Anyone that is a regular to Haunted houses knows that most stuff comes at you from the front or the back of the group. That's why the most scared will huddle in the middle. Non-regulars stick to the back. Honestly, you have to read the group to know which is which when they walk in.

First scare was right beside the curtain on entry. People's eyes were still adjusting when you come at them. I miss that. That moment after the person has been scared, and then they grin or laugh when they realize someone got them. I like those customers. I also like the ones that are not scared, but are clearly still having fun.

There are those one kind of customer, though, that made the whole dungeon not nearly as awesome.

The one that comes to mind when I think about them was when I worked in the back as one of the caged monsters. We didn't have enough volunteers to afford someone for the "First scare" spot. It went to the people at the cross to lead customers in the correct direction. Thus, my job was to yell and scream behind my heavy cage door as people passed. This ten or eleven year old boy had come through the Dungeon on his own. He acted like a pompous little brat that pretended he wasn't really scared.

When he got to my cage, and I jumped out from the dark to reach for him, he sneered, "You're not scary."

Bold words for a little shit that had backed up to the wall on the opposite side of the narrow hall. I glared at the brat, and decided he needed a worth while scare. I pulled up on the cage door for it to come loose from the hinge. It was not bolted. That's just how we got free from a 'locked' cage without locking and unlocking the person inside. I threw the heavy metal aside, and I ran at the kid, snarling like a mad woman. His eyes grew large, and he ran for the exit at the end of the hall. He completely missed the last two scare sections.

I was satisfied to have scared him, but when we were on break, everyone in the dungeon brought up the boy. No one likes the pompous customers that do a Haunted house for bravado, and just sneer at our attempts. It's supposed to be fun, but people like him don't make our job fun.

I suppose I didn't mind this "reliving a memory" trip. It was nice to be among friends and entertaining customers. Writing about it, however, is causing several twitches to other memories. Honestly, as nice as this trip was, it gives me a headache. I think I need a nap.

Life Badges

Scars are a funny thing. They're this physical reminder of a moment in our lives. I know there are lots of people out there that have scars that give them nightmares. Mine, however, generally lead to moments of stupidity. Some I laugh at. One I love retelling over and over. Being as pale as I am, a lot of those scars are unable to fully fade.

I know this seems out of the blue, but as I was typing the other day, I was looking at the scar on my right wrist. It's faded quiet a bit with time, but it's still there. An ever present reminder of the day I came face to face with my own mortality, and yet walked away with only the tiniest mark.

It happened while I was in Brazil for seven months. One of the host families I was staying with had an orchard in their back yard that had a tall brick fence around it. It sat, separated from the rest of the house, with only a tall metal gate to enter. I pity anyone who thought they were sneaking in there, as a pair of Brazilian Mastiffs roamed the entire place.

They were large, beautiful, brindle dogs, but I was warned, right away, not to go near them. I knew to respect a dog's space. There was a point when I was a child that I had been bitten on the nose by a Shih Tzu because I was trying to kiss it. It's actually a small fortune that one isn't a scar, either.

The orchard also had a picnic pavilion very close to the gate. There were plenty of days where the family would cook lunch out there, and eat. The dogs were always locked up during those occasions, and I had not thought anything of it. That day, though, I had been sick for most of the morning, but was starting to come around by 1:30-2 in the afternoon. I had missed lunch with the rest of the family, but I knew the Uncle was still out there doing clean up. I figured I'd go see if there were any leftovers.

I open the gate, having no idea that the dogs were loose. They had been hidden against the brick fence, trying to cool off in the shade. They were on their paws in no time. It was the sound of their nails against the tiny patch of concrete that caused me to freeze in place. My left hand was still firmly gripping the gate.

I breathe deep. I knew better than to attempt running from predatory animals. I stayed perfectly still in the space between the front and back yard. They were not aggressive when they approached. The smaller female held back, while the large male came up, and sniffed at my foot.

Now, I was wearing sandals. The kind that had small pieces of leather around the foot, and then crisscrossing shoelace on the top. The amount of exposed skin was in greater supply than the amount covered by footwear.

The male growled, and I twitched my foot just a little out of fear. I felt his teeth graze the top of my foot, and then I was being pulled to the ground. Yet, by some miracle, the male had grabbed the shoelace, and nothing else. When he pulled, I was able to continue balancing on my other foot because of my grip on the gate. While in this strange crouch, trying to pull my foot loose from the male's hold, I was eye level with the female.

At the time, I didn't realize how close I was to her because my main concern was the one that had a hold of me. She did not attack me, though. Instead, her loud bark boomed with hot breath on my face. I wonder... if I had turned and looked at her, she might have considered it a challenge, and attacked me. Regardless, her barking had signalled to the Uncle that the dogs were after someone. His shouting rang out, nearly drowned by the female's barking.

I saw him running towards us from the corner of my eye. He didn't make it to us, though. My shoelace had come untied. It unwound with such a force that the little plastic end snapped the male in the nose. As the male shook his head from the small sting, the backlash from me trying to pull free had me stumbling backwards. My hold on the gate causing it to slightly close as I righted my stance.

When I realized I was escaping, and needed to close the gate faster, I grabbed onto the side with my right hand. If I had held onto anywhere else, I would have made it out completely unscathed. As it was, the male realized I was escaping, and made one final lunge for me. His fangs had grazed me, enough to require two stitches, but he did not get a hold of me.

The Uncle had to put the dogs in their kennel. It was the house maid that examined the damage first, and lead me to the sink to rinse under water. The woman in charge of me while I was in Brazil was married to the doctor of the little town I was staying in. So, he easily stitched me up, and I didn't have to try figuring out how to use my health coverage because he and his wife already knew how.

A fellow exchange student, a boy from Mexico, had poked fun at me when the bandage finally came off, and it proved not to be that big of a wound. I don't care how big it was. I don't do well with pain, and the most sensitive spot in my body is on, and around both of my wrist and neck. So, yeah, I babied my wrist for a couple days.

It also took me a couple weeks to sort my thoughts, and fully understand exactly what had happened. I mean, it all happened in under a minute, or two. A lot could have gone wrong. If the dogs hadn't been near the concrete, I wouldn't have heard their nails, and stopped. What if I hadn't been holding onto the gate? What if the male had grabbed the leather of my sandal, or, worse, my foot? What if the female had taken advantage of my crouch, and went for my face?

At 17 years old, I had had a brush with death, and got away with only a minor scar. Sometimes, when I feel particularly low, I stare at the scar. I could be dead, I think. But I'm not. Sometimes, that's all I need to remind myself that I have a purpose. I was given a second chance. This tiny bit of discoloured flesh, and a memory.

One Terrible Tuesday Morning

Well, yesterday was quite the shit show. I had woken up dreading going to my painting class. It took several self-reminders that my professor had been the first to respond to Anita's e-mail asking how he could help, and that I had finished my project 2 last Tuesday to get me moving.

My Mum had even complimented the piece when she drove me home Sunday. I'm not sure what had brought it up in her mind, but she suddenly asked me, "So, what did you do with that picture?"

"What picture?"

"The one you sent me a picture of last week... what day was that?"

The one she had responded with a "cool" to, I thought. I hate it when she uses "cool" as a response, because she only does it when she's trying to fake interest.

"You mean my painting? I sent you the picture of it on Tuesday after I finished it."

Her eyes grew wide, "You *painted* that?"

"Yeah," I sarcastically smirk.

"I thought it was something you made on the computer."

"Nope," I felt a spark of pride make a hopeful course through me.

"Really? I seriously thought it was digital. Did you send it to Aunt Heather?"

She then proceeded to have me text the picture to my aunt. It's one of the best reactions I could hope for from my mother. No criticism, just awe. I'm still beaming at the thought of it. It was awkward painting my own face, and it'll feel self-centred to have it hanging on my wall, but I'm putting it up once I bring it home. I would give it to Mum, but it's too big for her walls. It would probably just end up on the shelf in the spare room with the other painting I made her for last Christmas.

Still, holding onto that memory, I decided that I could hand it in, and may just get a good mark... even with the past deadline deduction. My classmates, also, spoke highly of our professor. The few times I had been around him, I had to agree he seemed very chill and ready to help. Things had gone well with my other professors when I spoke with them. There was simply no reason at all to worry, I thought.

I had arrived to class early. Nearly ten minutes before it was officially supposed to begin. For anyone that knows me, such a statement would cause pause. I often joke that, since I'm never on time, I'll probably be late for my own funeral. In fact, I think I want to put it in my will so that it will happen. Something to give my friends and family a chuckle or two.

I nervously waited with the completed portrait in hand for him to finish setting out the paints. He gave me a neutral greeting, which only set me on a higher alert.

"This is your self-portrait?" he said as he walked over to his desk.

The sarcastic side of me wanted to say, "No shit, Sherlock." I mean seriously, it's a giant picture of my face. What kind of question was that?

Instead, I started to muttered, "Yes. I'm not really sure if it works for what we were attempting to do, though."

The last time I had spoke with him about the work-in-progress, he told me that I was blending too much. We were supposed to use solid colours on top of colours, referred to as "a painterly piece". This one in particular was based on a specific artist, but I can't remember that artist's name. I had stylized my self-portrait into a stained-glass version, and making the definition between tones and highlights using blending, instead of putting a darker or lighter colour on top. I tried to apply the other way as much as I could, later, but I'm not sure it perfectly represented the assignment.

I offer the painting out to him, but he didn't accept it.

"You're going to have to hand it in during portfolio week," he spoke matter-of-face.

My stomach lurched. To hand in a project during portfolio week is basically agreeing that you won't get better than a 50% on a piece. That was best case, too. I don't know if it was calculated by subtracting 50% from the final grade, or if the professor simple says, "it's good enough to pass", and gives it a 50%. Either way, to hand it in during portfolio week, especially since I wasn't sure if I had even followed the project requirement correctly, meant 20% of my final grade was in jeopardy. 40%, actually, since the same would need to be done for project 3, and I haven't even started that one.

I couldn't look him in the eye before, which is why I was pretending to be looking at his many ear piercing instead. After he had said that, though, I couldn't even look at him. Instead, I stare down at my artwork with disdain.

"What?" I barely breathed out a whisper.

He must have noticed the beginning of tears, because his voice turned sympathetic, "Well, it's way past due. The deadline is already closed."

My mind started to come undone. What about his e-mail asking what he could do to help? What about the disability accommodations? The little bit of hope I had been building up with help from counsellors and doctors was suddenly shattered at my feet.

I'm going to fail. After everything, I'm going to fail because I couldn't get my lazy ass to class. I won't be able to continue next semester. I won't be able to continue treatment with the people that had come to be a life line. I won't be able to afford staying where I am. I wouldn't even be able to afford a new apartment at a cheaper price. I would have to go back to Chatham, a failure once again. A college failure, which was worse than being a college drop out. And I would have to explain to my mother and family exactly how I had come to fail. I would have to hope that either my mother or my Aunt Heather would be merciful enough to take me in, or else I would be homeless.

All those thoughts circled out of control in under a minute. I was frozen in place, trying not to make eye contact with anyone. I didn't want to make a scene by crying. I didn't have the voice to even explain my thoughts, though. I was feeling trapped, and I just wanted to run, but I couldn't. I told myself I had to stand there, and be reminded that I had just screwed myself over, again.

Thankfully, the professor was kind enough to speak lowly, "Do you need a minute?"

I made quick, small nods. I'm sure I looked like my head was momentarily going into a seizure fit.

"Okay. Go get cleaned up, and we'll talk after. Alright?"

I nodded again, but I was already turning away from him. I hurriedly set my painting over my belongings where I had intended to sit. It was still early, so there was only a handful of people to see me rush out of the studio. I bee-lined straight for my favourite public safe-haven, the bathroom. Since it was before classes, there was someone at the sink, and two of the stalls were already taken. I shamefully hid myself away in the third one. The large handicap stall, of course. Part of me worried that a student might need it while I was in there, and I would be forced to come out.

Thankfully, no one needed it.

I stayed in there, tucked inside the stall with my back to the wall. I dare not sob or sniffle too loudly. As nice as it was to have someone pull me from my crying fits, I feel embarrassed. So, I'm left stuck between forcing myself to not be heard, and hoping someone will hear me anyway, and come knocking. No one did.

For over a half an hour, I attempted to sort myself out. The little reasonable voice told me not to worry. There might be a misunderstanding. Maybe he meant that he didn't have time to mark it until portfolio week. Maybe I should go talk to Linda or Anita, and see what my options are. If my professor's job required him to fail me, then maybe Linda and Anita could help me find a way to keep going, regardless.

That voice, however, was being swallowed up by doubt. That side was also being mean, and telling me I'm being ridiculous. Who cried over a teacher telling them they might fail? That wasn't even his exact words, anyway. What am I doing, making a scene like that in front of my classmates? I'm already not as close to them because of so much missed school time. I'm just making fitting in and making friends so much harder on myself. They probably all think I'm a whinny loser.

About ten minutes into my mental torture, another, angrier voice joined in. It wanted to blame my professor for this predicament. It shouted things like, "liar!" and "that traitor!". The voice was appalled that it was going to take one idiot to throw my life back into a mess. He wasn't being fair, and how could he say he wanted to help, and then throw me under the bus?

I hate being angry. It's such a dangerous and damaging emotion. Since most of my relatives and I have some serious tempers to us, I have grown up knowing, first hand, how giving into anger can turn a good person ugly inside. It only hurts everyone and everything, including the one that's angry.

That's why every time anger starts to add weeds to thoughts, I try to chop it down with logic. Reason reminded me that the professor was just doing his job. It was not a reflection on him. It's likely that the system in place did not give him the same wiggle room as the other professors. After all, his class only had a total of 4 projects worth 20% a piece, where the other classes had a couple more with varying grade weight.

I didn't feel any better by the time I had unlatched my stall. I just felt tired. Doubt wanted me to go home and sleep.

There was obviously no point being here today if all my projects have to wait until portfolio week. I may as well work on them on my own time, away from my classmates. I'm going to fail whether I'm here or not, anyway.

Anger agreed on leaving too, but only because it didn't want to be in the same room as that 'liar'. I didn't even want to go back to the class to get my belongings. My legs were shaking when I did.

I practised a convincing "tired smile" in the mirror after I used a cold compress to remove the heated red from around my eyes. It was just in case someone stopped to ask me if I was alright, or what was wrong. No one did, though I'm not sure if I'm grateful for that or not.

I did not look at any of my classmate's faces when I entered the room. The spot I had picked had been near the wall, so it was easy enough to slip in. Except the professor was in the way of my direct path, because he was helping another student with a question. I told myself to breathe deeply as I scurried around that table to my own, and gathered my things.

My reason stilled my flight, though. It told me I should, at least, be respectful enough to let him know I was leaving, instead of just storming out. He had asked me if I wanted to talk, after all. He wasn't a bad guy, and I didn't need to be rude. I waited. I used the excuse that I needed to get the paperwork about what was needed for our portfolios.

"Do you want to talk?" he asked again.

"What's the point?" I snipped. Oops... so much for holding back my anger.

"Okay."

Seriously? I had to remind myself that he was probably being respectful of my wishes, and not just being dismissive. Still, it was with a stiff walk that I followed him to the front of the class to his desk.

He didn't just hand me the paper and let me leave, though. He had to point at the line that said, "project 2. 20%".

"Alright, so you have project 2 done."

Clearly, since I did just put it back with the other project 2 paintings. With anger boiling just under the surface, I had considered coming back to class, and making a point by throwing it out, or ripping it to pieces. It was the fact that it was something Mum had complimented, and actually showed belief in my skill, that stopped me from acting out so childishly. Besides, I didn't need to throw a fit in front of the whole class.

I simply nodded.

"Do you know what project 3 is?"

One of the other student's version of project 3 was on the wall in front of us. "Like that," I pointed.

"Yeah. Do you have it done?"

"No." I snipped again. If it was done, I would have been trying to hand it in with the self-portrait.

He glanced around the class. "Okay. So, just have a look around at some of the others' examples."

Stop talking, already, anger silently urged.

I want to leave! Hopelessness added.

I just nodded.

"And do you know what project 4 is about?" he continued.

Reason chose then to point out he's clearly just trying to make sure I knew what I had to work on so I could do so on my own time.

"Not really," I admitted. I had been more concerned with 2 and 3 that I figured I would get to 4 when I got to it. I knew where to find the outline on our class online thing.

"Okay, let me go get you the rubric..." he trailed off.

Before he moved away, though, I hissed, "What's the point?"

Fucking anger.

I think he was getting fed up with my attitude, because his own voice grew a little colder. "The point is, you can still get a mark for it. *If* you hand it in on time."

That set me off, again. "If" I can get it in on time. Because the likelihood was, I couldn't. Not with one other project to finish before that. Though, why should I finish either of them if I'm just going to fail? It didn't pass me that that line was him scolding me for falling so far behind. Reason could no longer quiet anger.

On and on my thoughts reeled again. Rage was taking the lead, wanting to yell and punch a hole into one of the walls. I needed to rip into something, physically or emotionally, but I couldn't. I wouldn't let myself.

Drawing back, however, just returned me to my doubt, and fear for what my future held. I didn't want to go back to Chatham as a college failure. I can't go back to Ontario Works just to make ends meet. There was no logic to my thought anymore. Just pure, raw emotion. I was not going to let myself cry again, either. Not there, anyway. I had to make it back to the bathroom.

Holding back both reactions was causing my heart rate to soar, and my breath to chock. I was shaky. The last bit of respectfulness I could muster came out as a stuttering, "I-I... I gotta go. I... have to go."

I think he answered, but I'm not sure. I barely remember myself leaving again. I know I made it back to the bathroom, but I was gasping for air. I do remember the question, "what am I going to do?" playing over and over.

It took two minutes before reason made another desperate suggestion: go to Linda or Anita. Instinct agreed, and the next thing I remember is standing in the Counselling office.

Hot Tempered and Panicked

I had had these sorts of 'episodes', as I called them, before. They're incredibly rare, but they generally have a lasting impact. It happens when fight and flight kick into over drive, but I have enough sense to know neither is appropriate. It's forced to bottle and fester until it chocks me. A sensation made all the more difficult by sharp hiccup-sobs, and shaking limbs. Most of those times, my logical thought completely shuts down. I'm left confused, exhausted, and have to rely way too much on pure instinct.

The two other times that come to mind that these happened led me to hitting someone. The first was when I was in my grade 8 year. My sister, our friend, and I were playing on a snow hill in the early spring. School had just got out for the day, and we had a few minutes before we had to be home. A girl named Courtney, and her two lackeys, happened by us on their walk home from school.

Well, I'm fairly certain I've told this story once already.

The second time I remember having an episode was more recent. I was eighteen, and my sister was freshly sixteen. Throughout the last couple of months, our sibling spats had lead to fist fights.

There were a lot of factors in place that lead to this fight. Too much to really get into right now. The point is that we were fighting while also storming up an down the stairs. Mum was working at the time, and unreachable by phone.

At about the seven minute mark, Cam finally lost the last of her temper. We were heading up the stairs, again. She stopped at the top, and suddenly turn around to boot me in the stomach. My hand on the railing is all that spared me from falling back on the stairs, and likely hitting my head on the table dangerously close to the base. Like every physical fight we had done so far, that hit meant that attacking her was fair game. I charged up the last step, and grabbed onto her.

I don't know what happened from that moment until my sister was shoving me aside, and running out the door. I have, since, pieced the clues together, but I don't remember it happening.

I had punched my sister in her lip. Hard enough to split it against her teeth. Hard enough my knuckles were sore, and there was a small scratch from also hitting her tooth.

There was blood on the wall and our family portrait, because I had had her pinned there when I hit her. A bloody hand print on the wood of the sliding door that separated the downstairs levels from the upstairs ones. That was from when she was fleeing out the side door. There's still a prominent scar above her lip. She used to try covering it with lip piercings. Sometimes I feel guilty looking at it. I know she started it, but I should never of let my temper get the better of me. Thankfully, that was the last time she and I ever had a physical fight.

The point is, both of those occasions had triggered the same response from me as my encounter with my professor on Tuesday had done. I'm not sure what I would have done if I hadn't left when I did. I definitely would have been in a heaping pile if I had acted out violently.

All three cases though, I was shaky with adrenaline, crying, and having difficulty breathing. When I got to the Counselling office, I could hardly sputter out that I needed to speak with either Linda or Anita. Unfortunately, Linda was out for the day, and Anita would not be in until 11 o'clock.

The receptionist did take me to the back to a place called "the Quiet Room". It was a nice place, and when I had described it to my sister, she laughed and said it sounded like daycare. I mean, it practically was with it's teddy bears, happy pictures, and adult colouring book.

The receptionist sat down with me. She asked me if I was okay while she handed me some tissues. I can't remember if I responded with a deflective nod or a snarky answer. I was in the sort of mood that she could have gotten either. She asked me if I was having a panic attack. That question helped Reason break through the muddled up thoughts and emotions, and actually consider if that was what it was. I always identified it as "frustration" or "adrenaline" or, most commonly, 'an episode'. From what I know, however, those are exactly what make up a panic attack. Right then, far more than the other two times I mentioned, I was most certainly terrified. I had felt like I had just been side swiped, and I was back to no longer having any hope for my future.

I answered with a vigorous nod, and a stuttered, "yes."

She asked me if I had a technique in place to help me come down from it. Surprisingly, I did. Not because I had used it myself before. I knew it better for the fact it was what I often told others that I knew had anxiety to use. I had read once a grounding technique known as the 5,4,3,2,1 effect.

5 things you see.

4 things you hear.

3 things you feel.

2 things you smell.

1 thing you taste.

I stumbled over my words, trying to explain just that to this kind woman. By the time I got the point across, as matter-of-fact as I could muster, I was already starting to calm. As soon as I realized that, I decided not to do the 5 senses trick. I just started to think of as many random facts as I could. Which is a lot.

There's a reason my family refers to me as "The Walking Encyclopedia of Useless Knowledge".

After calming some, the receptionist helped me sign up for a triage counselling appointment. After she left the room, I snuggled with one of the teddy bears. I'm a sucker for stuffed toys. I put the bear back before the counsellor, Gillian (Jill), had come in to see me.

I have to give Jill credit where it is due. She got me talking, and calmed enough that I was able to leave the Quiet Room by eleven. Near the tail end, when I was verbally repeating my thoughts, she actually quoted my own words against me, because I was starting to ebb back into doubt.

"I know I've got a chance. I just have to keep trying."

Usually it's annoying when someone uses your own words against you. When she did it, though, I grinned. Touche, Gillian. Well played.

She did inform Anita about what happened. I also got to meet with Anita at 4 o'clock. I had forgotten she had arranged an appointment with me. She's now deemed that we meet every Tuesday at 4, though, so it's easier to remember.

Here's the kicker. During our meeting, Anita was geared up to send a message to my painting professor to help get to the bottom of this. I mean, I felt like I had been childish for "tattling" on a professor that was just doing his job. Both Gillian and Anita told me not to worry about it.

Then, to both our surprises, Gary had sent her a message while she was writing. It turns out that the reason my professor was washing his hands of me, and my late work, was because Gary had not spoken to him yet about my academic accommodations. For all he knew, my mental health excused my attendance. His other email was him offering to make it easier to ensure I come to class. There was nothing about how he was to grade me. According to Anita, the email from Gary said he (though I don't know if "he" was Gary, or my Professor) was super apologetic.

At the end of the day, it was a miscommunication problem. I can't blame my professor for that. On Tuesday, I was in a state that I didn't want to be anywhere near him. Now that it's Thursday, I feel better. I think I should be able to try again. I don't know for sure. I never know how I'm going to be until I wake up in the morning.

After all that, plus two other appointments, I came home,

exhausted, at 6 pm to my sister washing my dishes for me. I probably would have hugged her, except she's not the touchy-feely sort. Like I said, we're day and night about a lot of things.

 I grabbed my dish towel, dried, and put away what she had done for me. We talked about our crappy days, and I decided we should have sushi buffet as a happy finish to an awful day. It worked out, since Cam also wanted to stop at Walmart which is across the street from the sushi place. I was tired beyond belief, but that just resulted in my head drooping on the bus ride back home, and causing Cam to giggle. I didn't stop myself from dozing, since it felt good, and was making her laugh. According to her, I had started to lean towards a stranger two seats away from me.

 "I thought for sure you were going to snuggle with a stranger on the bus!" she kept teasing. I laughed along with her. I've said it before, but man am I glad I have a sister.

The Summer of '05

I met Nick Shepard at St Vincent De Paul summer camp. It was the year between grade 8 and 9. For me, that meant I was leaving the old school I had attended for ten years, to a new, and much bigger one. I don't remember a lot about how I felt towards the change. I do know that summer I was still sour about 'being rejected' by my grade 8 crush.

In all fairness, I know now how ridiculous it was to want to hang around him and hope he had more courage than me to ask for a date. Now a-days, I'll ask if I'm interested, and I think the guy is taking too long to ask me out first. Back then, I was a girl on the low rung of the social ladder with a thing for a nice, sporty boy who was perched near the top.

I went into an "all boys are stupid" phase, right up to the end of August. That was the year my sister was old enough for Mum to allow us to go to co-ed week, rather than one of the all girls ones. That ended up being the strangest week of summer camp I will ever remember.

For starters, my man-hating mode had led me to sit and draw instead of eyeing the boys with the other girls. Granted, I probably wouldn't have anyway because I was there to vacation, not ogle. This was apparently odd to my fellow fourteen-year-olds. I don't remember the conversations well, but I do remember one girl asking me, "Don't you like boys?"

"No!" I spat. I was hoping to stay far away, or show them up like I did as part of Scouts Canada.

There was a pause from my cabin mates, and then another girl asked, "Do you like girls?"

"Yeah..." I spoke as if it were obvious. Dumb ass me had been so innocently clueless that the question wasn't about if I think girls were cool, since boys clearly drooled and all that immature stuff we say about the opposite sex while growing up.

Instantly, the group of girls that had been sitting on and at the picnic table for Cabin 8 scattered. One even cried out, "Ew!"

Boy, that was embarrassing. I laugh about it now, since I'm now comfortable in my sexuality. But there was a time from about my mid-teens into my early twenties where I questioned if the reason I noticed other women so much might have an underlining meaning. I never experimented, but I did start to be more aware of where my thoughts went when I was "checking someone out" of either sex. I started to realize that a hot man would cause that nervous belly flutter, but a hot woman gets analyzed in matters of, "why the fuck is she considered hot?"

Further more, I could not stomach the idea of kissing another woman. Anything less than that, I already do towards my friends of either sex. Anything more, well, I figured this negative of a reaction was a good indication that I was not, in fact, bisexual. Which is a shame, because I've met some nice women through the ages that would make way better girlfriends than most of my ex-boyfriends.

Yet, I'm pissed to think that another girl in my place, one who was bi or homosexual, would have been ostracized from her cabin-mates that entire week. I get that a group of girls from 12-14 years old back in 2005 would not be mentally prepared, but it bothers me to think there are men and women out there that experience that level of shunning over something that's their business only. Especially if the ones that shun them is their own families.

But back to Mr. Nicholas Shepard. The quiet, specks-wearing boy from Cabin 3. Our cabins were assigned as buddy cabins. Thus, any activity we did was with the combined force of 8 and 3. I saw a lot of him that week. I still cannot say for the life of me what about him had charmed me out of my man-hate in under a week. Heck, it took me nearly two years to get over my first crush. I thought it would have been just as long for my second.

In a single week, I was doe-eyed, and in love. I think it was because we were both slightly to the outside of our respective groups. We came to actually camp, and enjoy it, while the others treated it more like a week-long speed dating special. Plus, I was the shy, pudgy girl that made it clear she preferred to do things for herself. He was withdrawn, and his glasses and braces gave him a rather geeky vibe.

That week, we were a pair of peas just shaking our heads about how immature our camp mates were being.

During our camp down time, we preferred to join some boys from Cabin 5 for a game that involved tossing a football between two teams. The one that caught it for their side, got to throw it back at the other side. By the end of the week, Nick and I knew who to team up with so as not to be tackled, and which boys would take turns. I think it was just my team being gentlemanly, seeing as I was the only girl that regularly played. Meanwhile, our cabin friends would sit at the picnic tables gabbing about whatever popular kids talked about back then.

The last night of co-ed week surprised me. Apparently, there was a dance. I should have figured as much, looking back, but I was used to the all girl camp routine. I'm not a fan of loud music, and people randomly screaming. It's why I detest concerts.

To add insult to injury, I had been to several dances before then, but I had never danced. I'm still uncomfortable with moving my body to music.

The last time I tried was at the grade 8 graduation party. I had started to sway a little bit, but some of the other girls pointed out I was actually trying to dance. Frightened because I thought they were going to tease me, and embarrassed to be pointed out, I ran. Not for a bathroom that time, though.

As for the camp dance, I tried to make the best of that night. Mostly, I shuffled around the hall by myself, hoping the night would end quickly. I was back to being shy, and a very small part of me hoped Nick would have the courage I lacked to ask me to dance. He didn't. In fact, we stayed away from one another for the first hour of the dance.

We did eventually sit down to chat. His older sister had approached me not fifteen minutes before, and told me that he liked me, but that he was painfully awkward. Thus, I ended the distance between us, and forced myself to keep shooting down any expectation of a dance that night.

There was, however, a boy from Cabin 5 that asked me to dance. I don't know who he was. We had hardly spoken to one another all week. I just remember that the football we had been throwing around during our down time belonged to him. And he was usually on my team.

It's possible he had liked me. I had not been among the number of girls drooling over his muscles. Still, as I sit here thinking about it, it's more likely someone put him up to it. I don't know who would have, or why. I can only really speculate with an eleven-year-aged memory. He was two years older than me. A huge difference when you're fourteen. He was strong and good-looking. So, why me?

By that point, I had found a bench, and had started up a conversation with Nick. Basically we were acting the same as the rest of the week.

Then the first slow song of the night started. I'm not sure if Mr. Cabin 5 had called out to me, or if I had just noticed him moving from the crowd towards us. That much bulk on a teenaged boy is hard to miss. He confidently outstretched his hand, and made a nod of his head towards the dance floor.

"Come on," he said.

I was terrified. I can still feel my legs shaking as I accepted the outstretched hand. As he led me to a clear spot nearby, I remember looking back at Nick. I don't know if I was pleading for him to save me, or if I was trying to convey an apology. I do remember that he had a look about him akin to that of a kicked puppy. Honestly, if I had known then what I know now, I would have enjoyed the dance instead of doing what I did next.

Cabin 5 and I had just set our hands on each others shoulders. The camp didn't allow hands on hips, and the camp counsellors went around with measuring sticks to make sure people were staying an appropriate amount of space apart. He led a slow spin, and I clumsily followed. We hardly made a full turn before two girls from my cabin came running up and mockingly shouting, "Aw!"

I could not handle it any longer. I let go, and ran for the bathroom. It was closer than running outside. There were two toilets. Not official boy and girl bathrooms with stalls. Naturally, both were occupied. I stood, paralysed, in the corner. It was a terrible hiding spot, and I knew I had just reacted in the dumbest way possible.

Gulping down my fear, I moved to the end of the hall until I could peek around the corner. The two girls from my cabin were on me faster than I could blink. They pulled me back to where I had been dancing, and Mr Cabin 5 was returning. Except, he was trying to wrestle Nick to his feet, and towards us. Nick held his own, but the poor skinny boy was a ragdoll to Cabin 5's strength. Maybe Cabin 5 did actually like me. I'll never know

I swear, Nick and I must have been quite the sight. I was about ready to dart back to the bathrooms, but that would mean shoving the two girls from my cabin. I could have. I was certainly much stronger than them. I stayed, though, because I really wanted to dance with Nick. We had just worked up the confidence for us to touch one another's shoulders when the song ended. I don't remember where Cabin 5 and my cabin mates had gone after that. I do know that the girls were bugging me for details about my night when we all finally returned to our beds.

They were disappointed to find out that we had spent the three hours just talking at our bench. To be honest, I was too. I think my thoughts were along the lines that if Nick knew I was interested in him and wanted to dance, maybe he would be up for it. By about the fifth or sixth slow song, however, I was comfortable enough to ask him instead of continuing to wait. He told me that he didn't really dance, said it was because of something private about his father. Having issues with my own father, I had let it be.

I know now that it was a blatant excuse. He's not one to up-front admit to being uncomfortable. He also has this mentality that he's a warrior surviving life's war. He's all about his excuses.

He had an excuse not to dance that night. A couple days later, even though we lived a forty-five minute drive from one another, I asked him to be my boyfriend through MSN chat. He agreed. We 'dated' for about a year and a half, only getting to see one another at camp the following year, and when his mother picked me up to celebrate his birthday. Then, during one of our phone conversations, he told me that we should not be dating.

"Well, my sister was told she was not allowed to date until she was sixteen. So, it's only fair that I wait too."

A load of bull. We were fifteen by then, and I was far from being his first girlfriend. Of course, I did not learn about the previous six girls until a couple years later. Despite his desire to end our relationship, I countered his excuse with logic. Instead of being truthful, he backed off, and we continued to date. I sorely wished we had ended it there. That however, is for another passage.

To Market

Do you ever have those days where, for no reason in particular, your intuition wants you to go somewhere or do something? With today being Saturday, December 3rd, I had intended to spend the entire day in the studio, working on my various projects. When I woke up, however, I had this inexplicable desire to find out when London's Western Fair district was having their Farmer's Market. Turns out, it was today.

Apparently, it's a weekly event. I knew there was a farmer's market there, but I honestly had no idea when it was open. Once I did know, however, I kept getting this tug telling me to go see it. It was 11:30 am by the time I finally caved, and went.

I got off the bus, and headed for the building, the smell of hot dogs on a bbq wafting through the cold morning air. I never did locate where the smell was coming from, because once I was inside, there was a plethora of other scents, sights, and sounds. The first floor was everything farm and food related. Butcher's shops and baked goods. Even a coffee bean place as soon as you get in the door.

I don't drink coffee (or eat anything coffee flavoured). I simply detest the flavour, but, for some reason, I love the smell of it. It's a fantastic thing to wake up to, without actually caffeinating my system. To walk into the market, and have that as the first thing to greet me, I instantly felt alert, and excited.

There's even live music. Beside the stairs was a man playing a violin. I would recognize the sound of one anywhere. They're one of my all time favourite instruments.

I found myself drawn first to a homemade bread merchant. There were two, but the first one I found was closer to the door when I entered. I was debating if I should grab one of the two roasted garlic bread loaves when a gentleman came by and bought them both. I figured that was a good a sign as any that I wasn't meant to get it.

The next place I stopped was a baked goods spot. The windows on the side I had come from had not held much to my interest. Cupcakes, cookies, and the other usual stuff that I could bake myself. Instead of walking away, I made the mistake of checking the other side. Cherry cheese cake... My pastry nemesis. I am a sucker for most sweets, but I do have enough self-control to turn away from almost all of them if I'm in the right frame of mind. I mean, when I'm stressed, people know to keep me away from candy, less I spend a small fortune. Today, though, I was having more than enough fun to pass by the sugar shop merchant with only a minor longing glance.

Cherry cheese cake, however... especially home-style recipes. I can't think of a time I turned it down. I love that sweet, soft cake so much, I get rather miffed when it's done wrong. There are two restaurants in Chatham that I know better than to order any sort of cheese cake from. This little spot, though, barely squeezed in beside the front door, and had some fairly decent cheese cake. Still not as good as my grandmother's recipe. I could be biased, but I will argue that it's likely because she uses orange juice in place of one of the other liquids in the cake. It gives it so much more flavour.

I bought my little slice of deliciousness, but didn't eat it right away, figuring I was only going to be in the market for an hour, tops. Except there was so much to see, that hour quickly turned into two and half, and almost $40 in spending. That is a small fortune when you're an art student who is already in some serious credit card debt. I still say it was well worth it.

I came upon the second bread merchant near the end of my trip. Their loaves were much larger than the other, for nearly the same price. Better yet, their roasted garlic loaf also had Parmesan in it. I had no idea what it was going to taste like when I bought it. When I took a small piece off while waiting for the elevator into my apartment, it was heavenly. I should have figured it would taste like the garlic bread you get with most Italian foods. I mean, it's right in the freaking name. Except, the garlic was more subtle since it's baked into the bread instead of being a spread.

My journey also led me to the perfect jam to go with such a loaf. There was a merchant that sold nothing but homemade jelly spreads. Some were your common flavours, like strawberry, blueberry, and peach. There were a couple of odd ones, though. The strangest being their new red pepper jelly.

It came in regular and spicy. I'm quite fond of my spices, so when the merchant offered a sample, my curiosity got the better of me. Boy, does that hit the tongue like a mouthful of fire ants. I found out after I had already lapped up a taste, and felt my tongue, and cheeks heat up, that it apparently has habanero flakes in it.

It's a combination of sweetness, and the hot kick to the throat had me scooping the last small jar. Lucky, too, because there was someone else just behind me, as I was leaving, who asked about it. I should go back next Saturday, and see about getting another one to give either my grandmother or my sister. Maybe one each, and call it a Christmas gift.

I should also see about getting another roasted garlic and Parmesan loaf to bring with me for the family to try with the jelly. I know Grandma would expect everyone to try some with her, after all.

Oh, and speaking of Christmas gifts, I found the perfect one for my mother. It's always difficult getting her a gift. Some years I do great, like with the heated bed sheet. Other years, the gift is set aside and forgotten. Last year's is a perfect example.

I had no money to spare towards treating my loved ones. I just couldn't get into the Christmas spirit knowing I would not have anything to give them. It wasn't until Christmas Eve that I realized I had paints and canvases, and set to work on a pair of paintings with the most detail I could do in such a short night. My sister's painting was a Dr. Who Tardis in the middle of the Antarctic snowfield. There was a wreath on the door, and lights wrapped around it while little penguins looked up at it with curiosity. The top of the painting read, "Happy Christmas". I had purposefully switched out the "Merry" for "Happy" because Dr. Who is a British show.

For Mum, she used to really be into otters. The year I made almost everyone hand painted ceramic plates, I made her a stained-glass stylized one with a pair of snuggling otters. It was in the China cabinet, until she "cleaned out the junk to make it look more organized". Now it sits in the closed off spare room. Last year, I changed animals. Almost everything decorative that she buys any more is owl related. I had a couple of little elf owls cuddled together on a branch. A great full moon shone behind them, and they were sheltered by a forest of painted pine trees.

The message on hers was, "Owl Love You, Forever", with a little pink heart designating the word Love.

It's also sitting in the spare room. At least that one is propped on a shelf so you see it when you go in the room. She says it's there because she's going to be painting the hallway and her bedroom, so she doesn't have anywhere to hang it. Yet, she's found places to hang some random artwork she bought during her trip to Australia. And the painting that her friend painted for her of the Sydney Opera house. Oh, AND the photo gift my sister made for her.

The picture is of a little Santa ornament resting beside this sweet "letter to Santa". The letter basically reads that she doesn't want anything for Christmas, just that her loved ones are safe and happy. It's adorable, and one of the more tender things my sister has done. I am jealous, though. She probably spent way less time taking the picture, and editing it, than I did painting those owls. Yet, her picture is hanging, year-round above the stairs leading to the bedrooms. Best part of all, there's a giant space of blank wall between it, and the first bedroom door. Big enough for two paintings, but she can't be bothered to hang the one.

I know it's not just me she does this too. If she doesn't like a gift, she tucks it away, and it's never mentioned again until she's cleaning. Then, if it's something she can get rid of, she will. She can't just give away the art pieces I gave her, though. Thus, they're sitting in the spare room. Out of sight, out of mind. Basically, I need to stop making her stuff for gifts. Even when I can't afford anything else.

Which brings me to this year's gift. I found it on the second floor of the market, where all the artisan crafts are being sold. It's four pictures in a frame. The pictures are of common objects making out the letters to spell "Home". Mum has a picture like it already, but hers says "Love".

When she hung up that picture, she went on and on about how interesting it was. Specifically, that it was random things creating the perception of letters, instead of actual letters. I think she was hoping my sister would use her photography skills to make two more for her... "Live" and "Laugh" to go along with her "Live, Laugh, Love" theme.

Maybe that's why she has such a large blank spot in the hallway wall. Well, now she has something else to put there to go with her "Love" one.

I did eventually get to school to work on my projects for about 5 hours, after the market. I think the side visit help perk up my energy that I was able to stay so long. As strange as it is to go on a whim like that, it really did help.

Broken-Hearted

December 5th, and I'm exhausted. I came to realize yesterday that I had misunderstood when and what portfolio week was. I thought it meant that I needed all of my projects and portfolios completed for their respective classes the day of those classes, starting Monday of next week.

Turns out, this is the last week to have everything done. We have to send in the portfolio (which is a bunch of paperwork about our different artworks) next week, but the projects themselves were due by their respective classes this week.

Needless to say, yesterday I panicked. It wasn't a full crying fit kind of episode. I just couldn't get myself to leave my bed. When I did, I was barely able to get myself to play Sims, let alone drink, or clean. In fact, I'm not even sure I had eaten yesterday. That may be why I'm exceptionally hungry today.

The longer the day drew on, the worse I felt. I was berating myself for not going to the school to get done what I could. I had about a dozen different ways that I was calling myself "lazy" for not attempting to clean. I felt horrible for my cats, who just wanted my attention. Aurora had to have cuddled up next to me at least four or five different times.

I decided I had spent too much time alone that day, and it was giving me too much time to dwell and worry. That's why, shortly after 5 pm, when I knew he would be available, I texted Nick. We seem to have this thing where we don't out right mention we want to visit until a couple hours into a conversation. I guess it's so we have the chance to mention if we already have plans. It helps me get a read on where his mood is at.

Yesterday, he was in just as bad a mood as I was. Except, he was sloughing his off better than I was on my own. He also already had plans, but said he "may" skip out early and come see me. I hate it when people say that. If you don't mean it, don't lead me with false hope. I did check in again around 11:30 pm just to talk.

You see, the relationship between us is so crazy and messed up. We use one another to stave off loneliness, and as a peer to talk through our troubles. And, yes, there is sex. It's just one of the things meant to make him feel better. It helps me too, because it's nice to feel wanted. I know it's all circumstantial, though. Karma had bit him in the ass, and he came crawling to me to make him feel better.

And I let it happen. No matter how much or how little is fake, he actually listens to me. He talks to me on a regular bases, and isn't judgemental about my weak spots. It's nice to not be alone. Especially in a city that is far away from my core family.

It does get awkward sometime. He wants to be around me to distract him from his own pains. Which, for him, is sex. He says every time he's here that's not what this is about, but considering that's how every visit ends, it's hard to believe otherwise.

Not that every time is solely from him. I have instigated it plenty of times as well. Even though I know I'll beat myself up about it later, I just need to feel something positive for a little while. I want to believe that I belong to someone. It's the closest I can get to someone wanting to be with me on a personal level.

I know all this adds up to a very sad conclusion. It means I've given up on finding love.

Once upon a time, I was all about finding my soul mate. That one man that completed me, who loves me for who I am, and who deserves all the love and loyalty I have committed towards the wrong sort. I'm a romantic. I believe we are all meant to find love.

Not fairy tale "love at first sight", bullshit. Real love. That old school kind of romance where you build each other up, and dream together. Where you can stand in a crowd, and still feel like it's just the two of you. Being able to cuddle and watch movies together without it needing to be about sex or heavy petting. When you know each others buttons, and can poke fun at one another. When you have those moments that you can't stand looking at them, but you know that, if they left, you would miss them more than air.

The kind of love you see in older couples that have already made it 20+ years together.

To be honest, I don't know if that kind of love exists in today's society. Not in my age range, anyway. Most of the time, you see couples that are all grabby and trying to inhale each other's tongues. That's not romantic. That's just making a statement to everyone else. Plus, if that's what they do in public, what does that leave for intimacy when they're alone?

I could just be reaching a point in my life where I think public displays should be much more toned down. Small touches, a peck on the cheek, or a shared look... little things to connect one another without screaming to everyone around you, "Hey, look at us! We're so in love, see?"

Then, when you're alone, cuddling becomes intimate. Play fights, and teasing, and listening just mean so much more. Which makes the more risqué stuff more special, and doesn't need to be all the time just to feel connected. After all, people age and slow down. Why build a relationship on a physical activity that will likely decrease with time, and general life?

To be honest, that's how the first three years of dating Nick had been. I was raised Catholic, grew up Christian, and had a very strong maternal desire since puberty. For me, sex was to be shared between husband and wife, and used for procreation. I stuck by that for a very long time.

Then, going on three years with my first boyfriend, it didn't take much for him to convince me. During a phone call, he told me that he worried that our relationship wasn't going anywhere. That we were "at a cease fire", were his words. I was terrified, thinking that he wanted to break up. I asked him what he thought would help. Intercourse was his answer.

The next Sunday, during his usual weekend visit, my sister was still asleep, and my mother was at work. I gave him what he wanted. I was a month short of being seventeen-years-old. At that point, I told myself we were expanding our relationship; like he had told me. I was already super loyal to him, but after that, I had figured he was to be my future husband. I did a lot for him. Started shaping my dreams to match his, but adding in my details. At the time, I had wanted 7-10 children. I realize now I would be happily content with 2 or 3.

When we were past the fourth year mark and inching closer to the fifth, we were acting as if we would always be together. At least, I thought we were. He is a very good liar.

The year I turned nineteen was crazy. My sister ran away from home. I was preparing to do a grade 14 year of high school to get the required courses to apply to the Registered Practical Nursing program. My Uncle John had married my Aunt Sandra in January. And I was also meant to be Nick's "plus one" to his cousin's wedding in June.

Being young, in love, and surrounded by people happily tying the knot, the future was all that was on my mind. I had once thought it was on his too, but considering the following events, it's questionable.

For some reason, my Grade 12 English class would get a bunch on real estate fliers. I often grabbed one to discus options with Nick when I saw him on the weekends. We had gone to view an old school house that had been turned into a three bedroom home. It was hilarious, because we went to the open house dressed in our medieval fair costumes; another event Gregor's Crossing regularly did in Chatham that I sorely miss.

All of it came to a sudden, painful reality check on a murky Wednesday in July. I know it was July, because my sister was back from running away. It was only for three weeks, but she was there. I thought it was strange that he came to visit in the middle of the week. He had been working at a factory for some time by then, so he didn't have the spare time to visit through the week. Just the weekends.

I had been doing something downstairs when Cam called out, "Hey, is that Nick's truck?"

I raced up the stairs in time to greet him at the side door. He gave a half smile upon entering. I knew his ques well enough to know he was nervous about something. He glanced once towards my sister, and then asked me if I wanted to go for a walk. Looking back, there were so many warnings, but I had been a love-struck fool that took his odd behaviour as him planning a surprise.

I do remember worrying that it was going to rain. He told me that we wouldn't be too long. I had wished the grey clouds would hold off as long as possible, because, by the time we had made it to the path around the creek, I had concluded that he was going to propose. I was shaking that I could hardly walk, yet grinning from ear to ear. I haven't the faintest recollection of what we were talking about as we walked around the bend near the baseball diamonds.

After nearly fifteen minutes of walking, I was starting to wonder what he was doing when he asked to sit on a bench near the bridge. I quickly plunked my butt down, and tried to remain calm. He sat down too, and he couldn't look me in the eye. His shoulders were hunched, and he was rubbing his palms together.

I instantly turned from excited to concerned, and asked what was wrong.

He told me, in almost a whisper, that he had been cheating on me with a girl he was working with. The sad thing was, I knew the name. For nearly a year, he had been talking about her. At the time, I had thought it was no different than him talking about CJ, his best friend. After all, the first time he had mentioned her to me, he told me CJ was interested in her, and he was trying to help get them together. He had told me about the movies the three of them went to see together. Another time, about a camping trip.

I had no reason to believe his loyalties would stray. To hear it from his own mouth was devastating, to say the least. To add insult to injury, he told me that, because he was cheating, we needed to break up. I still don't get that train of logic. It would have been too honest of him to realize I deserved far better, and was letting me go for my sake. After all, I later found out the only reason he told me was because CJ had gotten mad at him for taking the girl he was interested in, when Nick was already in a long-term relationship. Apparently, CJ had threatened to tell me. Instead of ending it with this other chick, he eliminated CJ's threat by telling me himself.

Which, from what I gathered from him over time, was also why he was ending it with me. He had figured that once I knew, I was going to dump him. It was better for him to be in control. He claimed that he was going to end it with both of us, but I don't think that's true. Honestly, I think he was just looking for a reason to end it because he couldn't come out and say it. I told him as much, citing the examples of wanting to break up because we weren't 16 yet, and that wasn't fair to his sister, and how he sounded like he was leading into wanting to break up if I hadn't offered sex. He denied it, of course.

I remember demanding if he had been sleeping with her. He said no, and I decided to believe him. I put him on the spot, asking why he would admit doing wrong, if he wasn't willing to try to fix it. I was so desperate at the time, I even said that I was willing to share. I realized how dumb that was later that night, but it had been enough to get his attention.

The next day, I sent him a message over Facebook telling him that he had one chance. If he wanted to work things out between us, he was to come visit on Friday like he usually did.

That I was willing to forgive him, but that meant facing up to my family (who can hold grudges far better than I can). If not, he was to get out, and stay out.

He told me he wanted to work it out. So, I made sure not to say anything to my grandparents. My mother already knew. Apparently, CJ had told my sister, and Cam had told Mum. She said she had told Cam not to say anything to me in case CJ was lying.

Again, things that I was told later on.

Since she knew, I figured it would be easier on him if we met at my grandmother's. It wouldn't seem out of the ordinary since I would sometimes be there on weekends along side my sister. Then I waited.

He would usually come to Chatham by 6 or 7 o'clock. When 10:30 pm rolled around, I got fed up and called him. The resulting phone call was an hour and a half long. Which gave my sister time to explain to my grandma why I was on the phone, crying, in the spare room.

A good friend of his family had passed away, and the funeral was Saturday. He said he wanted to work things out, but he didn't want to come over that night because then he would just be in a bad mood for the funeral the next day. He didn't want to slip up, and snap at someone for mourning the man since he accepts death as another part of life.

It's down right stupid, if you ask me. His funeral reasoning, *and* the excuse, I mean.

For someone that is diagnosed as "clinically depressed", even on my absolute worst days I am not suicidal. I have thought of death, and how much easier it would be to slip away. Yet, in my mind, doing such a thing would only give my pain to my loved ones. I don't wish that on anyone. I don't hurt myself, either; save for picking scabs (that's apparently an anxiety thing). Lastly, I would never use my mental health as a reason to hurt someone else. I mean, it took an extreme emotional break to get me to punch my sister. I don't wish death or harm on anyone. Not Nick, or my father, for that matter.

Well, I might wish an episode of explosive diarrhoea on Richard from time to time, but that's more to make myself giggle than a serious wish.

My will to not die resulted in an acceptance that death will happen one day. I don't know how, or why, or when, but it is inevitable for all of us. Which, on my good days, lets me remember to love deeply, be kind, and not worry so much. Someone might not be there tomorrow. I might not be there to apologize over a pointless fight. I never want to leave this world with people thinking I don't love them.

I'm not scared of dying. There will come a day I will meet the Grim as an old friend. I can hope it would be after I've lived a full life, but I know that not everyone is so fortunate. I understand that not everyone thinks this way. I know I've had my mortality placed in front of me the day I was attacked by dogs in Brazil. I get it, people need to mourn, because death is a big, frightening topic. It hurts a lot to loose a loved one.

Nick's mentality that people should get over it because death is coming for us all, anyway, is cruel, and selfish.

Further more, to use a man's death as an excuse to not face up to his mistake when he had already been given a second chance is even more cruel and selfish. Cruel to me, and a selfish slap in the face to someone that was supposed to be a really close family friend.

"Why didn't you call me, then?" I hissed.

"I did. I tried calling your mother's house," he countered.

"But I told you I would be at my grandparents' house."

"I didn't want to call there, because if your grandma had picked up, I figured she would have hung up on me."

"And I would have called you back! Don't you want to be with me?"

"I do..."

"Then why aren't you here so we can talk about it?"

Which led back to the part about the funeral the following day.

He did eventually agree to come. By then, I walked out of the spare room with a tear streaked face, and Grandma informed me that he was not allowed anywhere near her house. It frustrated me then, and I had to call Mum to ask if it was alright if Nick was over at her house so he and I could talk. She allowed it, but only because she was going to be in bed, and we needed to be quiet.

Now, though, I smile. It's the only time I can remember my grandmother getting angry for my sake. In her way, she was protecting me. She may blatantly favour my sister, or cousins (depending on whoever the youngest is around at that moment in time), but she does still care for me.

My conversation with Nick that night was short. After my grandmother, and sister's rants about him not being worth it, and me still very pissed off from him shoving my second chance in my face, I told him it was over. I don't remember what else was said, but I do remember him storming out the door. I remember heading to bed, feeling like a wreck, and Mum calling out to me from her bed.

She asked if he was gone, then, after I said yes, she asked if I was okay. I ended up curling up with my head on her side for about half an hour. I can't remember if we talked, or what we talked about. I know I would have stayed way longer, but Mum did have to be up for work at 5 am, and it was already well after midnight. She didn't tell me to leave, though, I just did to let her sleep.

The next time I heard from Nick was after I had a run in with his (at the time) step-brother, Robby. I was picking something up from the GME that Sunday. I knew it was a risk because Sundays were for Yu-gi-oh card game players, and, back then, Nick was a regular. Maybe I was hoping to see him to some degree.

He wasn't there, though, leading to Robby asking me if I had seen Nick.

"How am I supposed to know where he is?" I growled.

Robby was a clearly a bit taken back, "Well, he's your boyfriend..."

"*Ex*-boyfriend," I snipped.

I know the expression is "they're jaw dropped" to describe when someone is gobsmacked. Never once before, or since, I have seen it portrayed so literally.

"You guys broke up?" his voice cracked.

I kept my jaw clamped shut, because I probably would have started to cry otherwise.

"Why?" he pressed.

I took my purchase, and gave poor Robby a needlessly aggressive stare down. "Why don't you ask him?"

Apparently, he did. I got a message from Nick asking me why I was telling people we were broken up. Didn't I want to fix things? Yeah, basically the sneaky bastard turned it around on me. It was "my fault" we were breaking up. Since I thought I had made a mistake, I scrambled to try to fix it. For a month, it was push and pull. I kept trying to get him to choose; her or me.

He would hum and ha. Though I know now that I shouldn't have, I asked him what was so great about her. Why would he cheat on me?

He couldn't say for sure why he was drawn to her. I've figured out it was because she was playing him to get his attention. Doing cutesy things like doodling all over his water bottle. I'm sure she had given him some sort of physical gratification, too. He may have been telling the truth that they were not sleeping together, but intercourse is not the only thing a cheater can do.

He did, however, tell me that he started cheating because

he needed someone there more often. He was annoyed that I didn't have my license so that I could come see him instead of him always coming to see me. Plus, I didn't have a job.

I remember a debate we had. Not arguing. We didn't do that until the end. I realize now that that was a sign we were not properly communicating with one another. We were at his mother's house, and it was over me going back to high school for another year. Since I had gone to Brazil during my grade twelve year, I had already had to do an extra year to complete my Ontario Secondary School Diploma (OSSD). After that, I still didn't know what to do with my life. What I wanted most was to be a full-time writer, but until I published and gained readers, it was not a dream I could pay the bills with. Add in, taking too deeply to heart every time my mother tried to advise me of the negative sides of every career choice I had made. Honestly, it sounded, and made me feel, like she was disappointed in me for even thinking it. Thus, I chose to pursue the RPN program. It was the first choice I had made that Mum had great things to say, and was telling everyone, with clear pride in her voice, that I was going to be an RPN.

To get these courses required an extra year of schooling. On top of the two years I would be in college. He thought it was a waste of time. Never mind that I would have been making good money if I had completed the course. It was three years, and debt, that could be used earning money in some dead-end factory job like him.

I bristled upon hearing my lack of job coming up again. Honestly, those weeks dragged on. Listening to him compliment her, and belittle my choice to continue school. Hearing him complain about how I wasn't there for him, despite us calling and talking every day. After almost 5 years with me, and 1 with her, he just couldn't choose.

"It's like trying to choose between your children. How do you choose which one to save, and which one to hurt?"

He still says that when I bring up how he never chose.

August 26th, 2010... one day before our 5 year anniversary, and I had had enough. He wouldn't choose, so I made the choice for him. I wish I could say that was the end of it. I did try to move on those first couple weeks. Hurt and anger were good motivators.

Mum helped. She reminded me of all the things that made me who I was that I was changing because of him. Like my love of travel. He sees it as a waste of money. He's also extremely prejudice against immigration. Which leads to him being rather racist as well.

"We should all stay where we are, with our own kind. And if we don't like how our country is, we change it instead of moving somewhere else."

There are plenty of times his comments irk me. "You exist because of immigration, dumb ass." I would say.

"Yep. And I think that I'm an abomination."

Back then, my rose-coloured glasses led me to think he was just joking around. He was not as blatant about it then, either. He says it now, and it reminds me why I don't want a relationship with him. Nick can take his racial segregation concept, and shove it up his urethra (because that's more painful than the anus).

It's also very fortunate I have not fallen pregnant by him. The way he is trying to raise his daughter to be cold and unfeeling, "a warrior against a cruel world" he claims, disturbs me.

Oh right, I haven't mentioned he has a child now. The scarlet he had been cheating with popped him out one. He sent me a rose and a card in October (after our break up) to get my attention, since I wasn't responding to his emails. I thought it was a sign he was sorry, so I agreed to meet with him. That's when he informed me that she was pregnant. The baby was born June 4th. To think, he, very likely, spent our anniversary screwing this other woman, while I was a complete mess because of his doing.

A couple months ago, I went 17 weeks without a period. I've never been regular, but that was a record, even for me. I wasn't pregnant, but it brought up the topic of whether he would want a son or daughter. Either, he said, but he also made it clear that he would have liked a son more. He talked about how he would teach him how to chop wood, and clean a chicken for dinner, and other "manly" things (his word).

"And what if he doesn't want to do those sort of things? What if he's into dress-up, and dance?" I teased.

"It's fine when he's little. I played dress up with my sister all the time."

"What about when he's older?" my tone was far less teasing.

He shrugged, and laughed, "Then I'm gonna have to knock some sense into him."

There was a different conversation, during the legalization of gay marriage in the US, that he and I talked about what he would do if his daughter ended up liking women.

"I would have to disown her," he stated matter-of-fact.

Knowing how much of a sense of humour God has, I'm fairly certain one of Nick's children is going to end up part of LGTB. Probably his daughter, since he's fighting so hard to get her back. That would be the kicker, having to choose if he stands by or disowns the child he's been trying so hard to be apart of her life.

I remember why I was pushing Nick away so much after his girlfriend took off with their kid. He wronged me, held me on a string even after our break-up, and he had apparently moved on with his new girlfriend. Even now, he didn't choose me. He's with me because he needs someone there. Just like how I feel like I need someone.

I don't love him. What I was in love with was the affection, and the man he pretended to be. I have no reason to hold onto him. I owe him nothing. Though he's said he is sorry for his actions, and that he realized how loyal I had been all along, I can't take him at his word. He says he's willing to talk to my family about his transgressions, but I won't let him. That would mean admitting to my family that I'm being a fool.

Granted, they already know. I told my sister and Sandra. My grandmother has seen us out in public, and Mum went through my phone the one time I forgot to delete my messages to him (Thankfully it was just a "Happy Birthday" message). Grandma hasn't said anything, though, and Mum can't say she knows without admitting she went through my phone. She doesn't know that I know because of my phone's history. She's been trying to slip me up with random questions, though.

Thing is, I have been ready to let him go, and fully move on for over a year now. Ever since he was dumped, and I finally got to see him with a few more years of wisdom to me. I don't want him in my life. But I don't think I could handle losing the company he provides me. It's nice to have someone to play board games with, go for sushi, and spend hours debating various fandoms.

I just wish we could be friends without the 'benefits'.

My Familiars

I officially love Fanshawe, far more than I ever did St Clair.

I'm also fairly biased since I chose to go to Fanshawe for the course I wanted. The course is stressful, but fantastic. On Monday I was able to knock out two projects in the same day. One for my 2D and 3D media, and the other for sculpture, so that I could add it with my classmate's projects in the hall H display.

The media one involved a large plaster tent, and two feet sticking out the flap like in cartoons. Those damn feet took me an hour a piece to sculpt out of wet clay, but it was well worth it. The end result was adorable. I took pictures of the completed project. I had started that day thinking I still had to paint the tent, but the professor told me it was supposed to be white to project a film over. Then, since I didn't need it anymore, and it was way too bulky to bring home, I smashed the tent, and took the feet home.

I'm probably going to do the same thing with the sculpture piece. We had to do a panorama scale with a found object inside a setting that it would not normally be found in. Someone in the other class had done a large plaster sculpture of a milk carton pouring into a smaller one. It made me decided that my found object would be a milk carton, since I had some at home in the fridge. Which led me to think of a dairy farm.

Thus, my panorama was a barn and field with cows, and a random chocolate milk carton. The two cows were a pain in the ass too. First off, they're about two inches long. The one is resting, and the other is grazing. I couldn't seem to get the back hoof to sit right on the resting one. The grazer looked more like a skinny hippo, thanks to it's legs being too chubby. Seriously, how does that much fat balance on four spindly legs? No wonder they look hilarious when they run.

Once the little suckers were painted (and lost both their freaking tails in the process), I couldn't have been prouder. They are actually super cute. A lot of people were saying so before when I finished the basic sculpt of the resting one, but I didn't believe it until they were finished. When all is said and done, I want to take a big heavy stick to the barn. As for the cows, I'm cutting out a block of the foam that makes up the base, re-wrapping it with green tissue paper, and sticking them to it.

Granted, I will need to find a spot to put them where the cats aren't going to get them.

Speaking of cows, there was one at the school today. A small grey one in a petting zoo as part of a two day "calming zone". There were also some goats, a sheep, a shaved down alpaca, and one fluffy grey chicken. Man, I thought I was having a bad hair day.

Oh, that reminds me. So, there is a rumour for college students that, if you don't have time for a shower, do a quick scrub with a wash cloth, and then use baby powder to get the oil our of your hair. Well, it works, but let me tell you...

Baby powder on your mattress to help remove odours and help with sweat stains... great idea.

Baby powder in medium-short hair... bad idea. Very bad idea.

It stuck to me all freaking day. Even now, at 11:30 at night, I can run my hand through my hair and shake out fucking baby powder. Of course, it's completely obvious. There is clearly white powder on my scalp where my hair is parted. Plus, I now know what colour my hair will look like once I start to go grey. If I do, anyway. Even when Grandma forgets to dye her hair, the greys are not that noticeable, and she's in her mid-60s.

Of course, I should be looking more at the other side of the family since I got all the light genes from them. Including the auburn blonde that had mixed with my mother, and grandmother's dark brown.

So, yeah, if you are in a hurry, and have no self-shame, baby powder is a great way to get the oil out of your hair, and smell fresh all day. Thank you, Nelly, for suggesting that. Was definitely worth the laugh.

Nelly is Renae, my good friend from high school, by the way.

My classmates are such good sports about it too. Someone had to have noticed, but not a soul said a thing. I even got two hugs today! One I gave to Kennedy because it was her birthday. The other was from Maggie, before she left for the day.

Oh, and Renee (My classmate) gave me a hug before leaving class yesterday, too.

I talked to my painting professor today. I mean, it took me until almost noon to work up the nerve to go anywhere near the school. As soon as it was just him in the studio, I went up to him with my head low, but still meeting his eyes.

"Sorry about last Tuesday," was the first thing out of my mouth.

"It's okay. Don't worry about it," he said with a kind smile. He was then straight to business, explaining what I still needed to complete for my last two projects, and what research was to be included in my portfolio. I wish I had been to more of my painting classes. While I was working on my project 3, my classmates were relaxing and making jokes with him. I see now why they say he's incredibly chill. He really is a cool guy. I don't know why I started avoiding his class to begin with.

Scratch that, I know exactly why. I was getting overwhelmed from my classes. Couldn't get myself to leave my apartment for a couple days. Suddenly, I'm behind on everything, and missing more classes. Then, when I am in class, I feel like an outsider among my peers because I had missed so many classes. Which caused me to be even more uncomfortable, and start to freak out that my moving had been for nothing.

Vicious cycle, really.

Which makes me so much more glad I recognized I was falling into one of my self-destruct cycles again, and reached out for help. Now, I have a whole group of people to back me, and keep me on track. I know now that I'm not being lazy, or stupid, or foolish... not on purpose. There are going to be days I feel fantastic, and can face the world with my head held high. On the other side of the scale, there are going to be days I just want to hide and cry, and pretend nothing exists outside my safe little bundle of blankets. The thoughts and feelings in my head are normal. They're okay. Most of all, the mean ones are liars.

On Sunday, they told me I was going to fail everything.

Today, I have hope. Tomorrow, first thing in the morning, I'm heading to the studio to finish up my last sculpture. Then I'm going to continue working on painting 3. Thursday, I'm going to do media 6, and wrap up painting 3, if I haven't already. Leaving Friday to create my last media project in time to hand in for final marking, and the weekend to do my last painting project. I have the time to do it all.

Better yet, I also have a couple hours to spare so that I can go back to the "calming zone". I might actually get a cup of hot chocolate, and a free massage, this time.

I'll have a longer look at the craft stuff, too. I think I saw a station for little felt Christmas ornament doll things. I know the other spot was colouring pages, though. I think I'll skip that one again. I have an adult colouring book around here somewhere.

If I can, I may scoop a round of N64 Mario Kart. There was a whole row of video games. Sadly, the only one I was really interested in playing was preoccupied.

Saving the best for last, I want to go back to the puzzle. The woman at the station had been siting with the box closed and to the side. Apparently, I had been the first person all day to approach and ask to do the puzzle. In 40 minutes, the two of us had made a lot of progress. So much so, we were allowed to have the entire little table wheeled to the back so that we can go back to the puzzle, first thing tomorrow. I'm very excited for that.

Mum and I used to do a lot of puzzles. This was before we had birds which collect feather dust, and poop on the pieces. It was not uncommon for the two of us to randomly come home from whatever we were doing, and just sit at the table in the front room for hours. The largest one we completed was 2,500 pieces. We had been working on one that was 5,000, but then we needed a spot for the rabbit cage turned bird cage for our disabled cockatiel, Trooper.

I was okay with the birds taking up the puzzle spot. I find animals are great for helping me stay balanced. On some of my low days, my two cats are either cuddling with me, or insisting I get up to feed them. It makes me feel far less alone.

Funny enough, I didn't have a cat when I initially moved out of my mother's place. I had a dog. Thing is, he got depressed going from a large house with two other dogs and a big backyard to run free in, to my bachlorette. He ended up moving back in with Mum.

Before that, however, I came to realize I missed having the company of a cat. So much so, I could actually feel my mood dropping. I decided that if I was going to get a cat, I was going to adopt from the shelter. I had been into the OSPCA before looking for a lost animal, or bringing in the odd, injured one to find out what to do with it.

Yeah, my sister and I were THOSE kids that would bring home wild animals that were injured. Mum still tells the story about when I brought home a garter snake that had had its tail nicked off by something (assumed to be a lawn mower). Mum hates snakes with a passion. I had learned from Nicholas to understand, and respect them. I've had my picture taken holding an adult boa when I was about 11 or 12, and a very heavy anaconda when I was about 23 years old.

Of course, Mum is just as bad about rescuing animals.

For the record, no, the OSPCA does not take in snakes, squirrels, birds, or field mice. At least, the Chatham one doesn't.

The Chatham OSPCA isn't very big. It's a very tiny entry way, with the desks squeezed together on the left, and a little room with cages on the right. My previous experience had taught me to not look at the cages in the front. Usually because, if I did, I would want to take all of them home. Far away from those prison cells. This visit, though, I should have looked there right away. It would have saved me, and Aunt Heather, two hours.

They ended up taking me to the back room (past the desks) where the cats were kept. I fell for each of them right away, but I was stuck between three toms. A large, brown tabby, a year old black cat, and a friendly, old orange tabby. You could tell that all three of them were starving for a home. I felt horrible, because I didn't know which one to take. I did narrow it down to the two tabbys. I figured the young black one was practically a kitten, and more likely to get adopted anyway.

A worker took me to a play room, and brought each boy in one at a time to see if either of their personalities outside of the cage made it easier to pick. It didn't.

The worker hummed, "Well... have you met Buttons?"

"Who?" I asked. I thought I had met all the cats in the back, and I couldn't remember any of their tags reading "Buttons".

The worker leaves the room, and then comes back in with this shaved down, faded calico. She had just been spade the day before, and so had a cone around her head. She was set down, and instantly came to me for attention, despite two other people in the room. She was a talker. She seemed to be telling me her entire life story as she curled onto my lap, and stared up at me with her big eyes.

I knew immediately she was the one.

I learned that she had been from an animal hoarder home. She had not been well cared for, because she had arrived full of tight to the skin matts. Thus, she was completely shaved down. You can tell she's not used to being brushed, because she bites the comb every time I come at her with it. Granted, she likes the sheer even less. Thankfully, I had learned from grooming Momo- a cat that took a chunk of my heart with him to Heaven- how to pin a cat down to shave them when their fur is too long.

She was about a year and a half, and had come to the OSPCA pregnant. Unfortunately, all the babies had been still born. They had her fixed as soon as they could to put her up for adoption. Which just so happened to be that day.

I was not sure about the name "Buttons" though. Sure, she fit the phrase, "cute as a button", but her personality was that of a chatty princess. She had walked into my apartment as if knowing she would rule the roost. Never mind that there was already a dog living there.

Being a bachelor apartment, the only comfy furniture I had was the bed, and the kitchen chairs. She, of course, jumped up and plunked herself onto my pillows almost at once. Her dainty walk, sassy attitude, and sweet little chirps all made me think of a high class lady.

I didn't just want to call her "Lady" though. It makes me think of the clueless protagonist in Disney's *Lady and the Tramp*. After asking for suggestions, it was Cam that suggested "Cleopatra". Thus, Lady Cleopatra... but I call her "Cleo", for short.

The other little hairball came along three weeks later. For

my family, I fabricated a lie about bringing the dog out to have a 4 am dump, and, while I was throwing it out, I noticed this poor little kitten behind the dumpster. The story continued on with me bringing him back inside, and then spending two hours trying to catch the semi-feral hiss pot. I guess that at the time, I was worried, even though I had my own place, Mum would tell me to take the kitten back if she had known the truth.

The real story is, Kev lived a short walk from my apartment, and I had gone over to hang out. He lived with another friend from high school, Victor, and Victor's girlfriend, Brittany. The two of them owned a pair of cats that were never fixed, so there ended up being three little babies. I had forgotten about Kev telling me about the kittens until they were running around the entrance hall. That night was the first time I had come to visit since he had moved.

After my surprised, "Kittens!", Victor had laughed and asked if I wanted one. I knew I shouldn't have, since I already had two animals to care for. Still, I couldn't resist.

While I was there, the first kitten I had seen was a tortoiseshell they had appropriately named, "Badger". The spunky little spit-fire had captured my attention, but she couldn't care less about me. Victor informed me that they were keeping her, because she had a prolapsed anus, and would need medical treatment.

That left the tabby male and torbie female kittens. Once again, it became a case of the cat choosing the human. While I was watching Badger take down her slightly larger brother, their sister decided my lap was a good spot for a nap. She stayed with me for most of the night while we all watched TV. Occasionally she would become alert just enough to twist a funny way, and purr up a storm. Then she was out again.

I can't say much has changed there.

They agreed to let me take her home that morning (yeah, we had all stayed up all night to binge watch a weird show). It was a half an hour walk to my place, so they had given me a large box to carry her in. She had been good for the first 20 minutes of the journey. Then she decided my fingers were an excellent toy. 5 minutes from my door, and she figured out how to pull the box top in a way that allowed her to stick her little head out into the morning air. I can still see her bright curious eyes with the early dawn light shinning down on us.

My aching fingers wanted to name her "Athena". I still kept it, but as her second name. She was called "Aurora", after I learned that was the goddess of the dawn from the same theology that Athena comes from. She's been my snuggle bug ever since. I mean, really into snuggling. I've never known a cat that likes belly rubs, but apparently she does.

Honestly, my girls have been my world, and help keep me sane when I've no one else to talk to. Though I'm not sure if I can be considered sane since I sometimes carry a conversation with Cleo. Speaking of, the princess wants attention, and I am ready for bed.

Overcoming Weeds

December 8th, 2016. It's a quiet and cold Thursday. A nice sensation after such an emotional roller coaster this week. Of course, that also means my day is fairly dull too. I had gone back to bed three times already since 5 this morning. It was the combination of a certain little hairball (Aurora) purring in my ear for attention, and the fact I shouldn't waste today by sleeping, that finally got me to my feet.

I'm not sure what to do with myself. I feel like I have a little energy in me to be productive, but I'm not sure if this should be utilized working on one of my projects, or getting those damn dishes done. There is also a strong part of me that wants to use this spark towards writing my novel. I've been away from it for several weeks now.

Cleo seems to think I should use it snuggling her, as she's now making it very difficult to type.

I'm writing in this journal, instead because of something I remembered while trying to go back to bed. It was one of the less pleasant trips down memory lane this time. Grade 6 was a changing year for me. It was the year I started writing. The year after I had been brave enough to approach a strange boy, resulting in my first friend in a very long time. Yet, it was also the most awkward, for that was the year puberty charged in.

It meant that I was the first girl in my age group that had to start wearing a training bra. I hated it, and the constriction. By now, it's par for the course, but I still choose not to wear one when I can help it. There were a lot of days that I would go to the bathroom to slip it off, and then hide it in my backpack. My mother will be the first to remind me of that whenever she talks to friends who's daughters are just starting their own hormone Hell.

The moment I remembered was during one of the days I had kept the damn thing on. I was at my locker, squished between others also trying to get to theirs. I assume we had just come in from recess, because the small halls required us to bring classes in one grade line at a time. During the warm weather, that meant plenty of students would misbehave just so we would stay outside longer. Even if it was in line. In winter and spring, it was the complete opposite.

My fellow classmates and I were taking our turn to scramble to be ready for class when grade 7 came in behind us. Actually, now that I think about it, although I did have my first period at 11 years old, in grade 6, for this to happen, I would have had to have been in grade 5. The 7s and 8s were in a different hallway, and thus, a different line.

Regardless, I was at my locker when a girl from a year older than me had suddenly reached out, and snapped my bra strap through my shirt as she passed. Since I was constantly on guard throughout elementary school, I had fast enough reflexes to whip around and pinpoint the culprit.

I know I had told a teacher. That was my go to at that age. I don't remember if or how she was punished though. I don't think she was. It would have been too easy for her to claimed it wasn't her, and how could I know for sure if my back had been turned? But I knew it was her. I had already been turning around the moment I felt a hold on my bra. She had not been given the chance to fully snap it on me because I had moved away. I saw her hand quickly drop to her side. I glared into her eyes when she continued on with her class line, and she was wickedly smirking back at me. The sheer hustle and bustle of everyone shuffling around in the compact hallway had worked to her advantage. There was potentially one hundred witnesses between the four grades that took up that hallway. Yet, not a soul had seen.

She knew, and I knew, and that was the point.

That unwelcomed reminder is one of few I haven't been able to counter with a technique I developed about two years ago.

Whenever a random memory of something bullies did or

said pop into my head, I think about how I would react to it now. It creates this false memory to compare beside the actual one. It's meant to show me how much I've changed and grown, boost my confidence, and not let old wounds haunt me. It's been quite successful.

One example was a memory from Grade 7 year. I was in the middle of French class with this vicious little bitch, Petunia, sitting behind me, and, the worst of my bullies, a boy named Ryan, in the desk across the space to my right. Luckily, to my left was the window, and the desk ahead was empty, so it was just the two of them.

Huh. Funny thought. I'm very picky about where I sit when I enter a room. I find myself most comfortable when I'm near a wall or window. I mean, despite having an entire couch to myself, I sit at the one farthest from my door that's also closest to my window. It had caused me some issues in high school, but it's still something I deal with. I wonder if it's an old instinct to ensure I'm not surrounded at any time?

Back to class, we were doing open study, and the two of them were teaming up to taunt me. Probably trying to distract me since I was easily zooming through the work, and they constantly had to ask the teacher for help. I don't remember what they were saying. I do remember I had got fed up, and rose my hand to get the teacher's attention.

Ryan mockingly pretended he had been insulted, and quickly rose his hand as well. Petunia was at my back, whispering that I was such a tattle-tale. I decided I was going to go back to pretending they didn't bother me. Except, my hand was already up. I had to wait for the teacher to come around, and then pretended I had a question related to the work. When she had finished "assisting" me, she had turned to Ryan's raised hand.

"Anita called me a name!" he blurted out, gaining the entire class's attention.

Before I fully registered what he was doing, I was already

defending myself. "No I didn't!"

"She did too. I heard her!" Petunia added.

"I did not!" I pleadingly looked up at the teacher. "I swear, I didn't."

I think the look on my face, and the two of them looking too giddy for someone that was 'insulted' had been my saving grace. Madam told Ryan and Petunia to ignore me, and I was told to pay attention to my work. It was the only time I remember a teacher scolding me (for something other than not doing my homework), and I hadn't even done anything wrong. Apparently, that deeply affected me.

The false memory starts just after Ryan falsely accuses me. I had considered calling him a name, so that's what he told the teacher was true, but I find it more satisfying to call him on his crap.

Instead of reacting, I look at the teacher, and patiently wait for her to ask me the same thing she asked every one of my bullies when I reported something they had done, "Did you?"

Imaginary me shrugs, "Hey, I'm as surprised as you. What *did* I call you?"

I figured the turn around would have pissed him off. Either he would trip up, or he or Petunia would blurt out "my" insult. It would have been hilarious if they had both spat one out at the same time, and really dug themselves a hole.

If either of them did say something, my new response would have been as sarcastic as possible, "Really? Wow, I didn't think I was capable of such language. Damn, I should really go sit in the hall for that. What do you say, Madam?"

I imagine that would have made the point that I was being falsely blamed while turning the bullying back on the bullies.

Now, every time that memory wants to pop up, I have my false one to beat it down. It's been a long time since I've felt bothered by it. As well as several others. I think that's why all the childhood bully non-sense doesn't leave me broken and in tears at night. It's easy to just shake my head, and remember that I was still a child at the time. Adult me would handle things way differently. Adult me is also very much a sarcastic asshole when I want to be, so I've got a fair arsenal to fire off when need be.

I knew this self-reflection thing was making a difference when I finally opened the Pandora's box of my childhood, and came to accept it as part of my past.

I have rather eccentric ideas. It works wonderfully as an artist, but as a child, I did a lot of odd things. I can control most of those impulses now as an adult. Save for the occasion something blurts out that my family teases me over.

The one that had put me in the lime-light as a main bullying target, was that I used to chase and bark at anyone that had come to bully my friend. I had, quite literally, pretended to be a guard dog. I'm not sure why younger me had first done it. I assume she continued because she thought it was fun. After all, the older kids were no longer picking on my friend, they were laughing and playing with me. By the time I realized they were laughing *at* me, however, the damage was done.

I had been slapped with the title of "Dog-girl", and was forced to carry it well into high school.

The other kids didn't want to be around me because I was weird. The girl I had been defending had to move away, and thus I was friendless. For the longest time, I even hated dogs because they reminded me of what I did. I eventually got over the hating dogs part, because I have a deep love for all living creatures (even humans). The Dog-Girl title, though, haunted me. The last time I had heard it was in Grade 9, but there were still points well into my 20s where I would remember, and cry.

That overwhelming fear, and self-loathing nagged at me. Any time I told myself I was normal, and that I had real friends that liked me for me, a cruel voice would say, "Oh yeah? What about Dog-Girl?"

I refused to bring it up, or talk about it to anyone. Not family, friends, or counsellors. I wouldn't even let Cam mention it. She seemed to realize what a sore spot it was, and never used it against me. It was tucked away inside to become a vast weed because I could not face it.

There was a time I was playing some catch game with my cousin, Madison. She was maybe two or three at the time.

She would throw her bunny toy, I would go get it. I would, then, put the rabbit's face into hers so it could 'kiss' her, as I playfully told her not to lose him again. Which, of course, she would throw it, anyway. We had carried on like this for a good twenty minutes. The room was filled with her howling laughter, and I was grinning ear to ear. My Uncle Aaron, Aunt Kristen, and Grandma had laughed every time Madison did.

Then Grandpa made a comment that I was playing fetch like a dog. Instantly, the game was ruined for me. Madison didn't understand why I had suddenly stopped playing. I couldn't even get myself to come up with a new game for her. Twice she threw the bunny again with a half-toothy smile.

The first time, I returned it to her, and firmly said, "no more."

The second time, I left it laying on the floor, and decided to go upstairs away from my family. Which left Uncle Aaron attempting to explain to the toddler that the game was all done. Like I said, that was about nine or ten years ago. Well after I had stopped hearing that name, yet still fresh enough to completely ruin my mood over a simple, harmless comment.

Then, last year... not even a full year ago, in fact, my mind had to start digging deeper to attempt to bother me with memories for my younger school days. The only one it had left was Dog-Girl.

The obvious counter was that I certainly would not do something like that now. It didn't help to think that though, because I have no idea what possible changes would have happened if I had never done that. I can't say who I would be if I hadn't drawn attention to myself to be bullied.

When I started to get upset, I remembered something else. I used my growl that I had perfected back then to entertain children; as a small spook before going in to tickle them. Sonia and Dean love it. It's a game to them. Just as Dog-Girl had started as a game for me... because I had been seven-years-old when I had done it.

Just like that, I couldn't change the memory of my action, but I had a solid counter for every memory of someone using that name to get to me.

"Seriously? You're going to bring up something I did when I was seven? Should I call you Shit-Drawers, or Nose-Picker because that's something you did as a kid?"

"I was seven. Have you talked to a seven-year-old lately? They're rather imaginative, and filter-less."

Suddenly, I didn't feel like such a freak. I had been a normal child, doing normal child non-sense. I also realized that if I had done such a thing towards my own age group, they would have thought it was hilarious, and played along. The reason I was bullied for it was because it was around older kids. Ten-year-olds, to be exact. An age where doing such a thing was dumb, and weird. They were the ones to give me that name. Being older, which instantly made them cool to my grade-mates, is what got me shunned.

For the first time since then, I was able to accept Dog-Girl. There is a part of me that still lightly twinges as I write this. A voice saying, "No, don't write that! What if someone reads it? They'll pick on you about it for sure."

Yet, now, I have a braver voice that says, "If they have to resort to something I had done almost twenty-years ago, as a *child*, it's clearly because they are desperate for *anything*, to pick on me about. Which is a sign that they have their own issues to work out."

It was my last, painful secret to understanding my past. I wasn't ready to accept it before. With each passing day, however, I'm able to understand it more and more. Maybe one day I'll have the strength to take out that fucking weed completely. When that day comes, I'm bringing a dragon to burn it to the ground. Much more interesting than an imaginary flame-thrower.

For now, I don't have to cage up Dog-Girl anymore. She's free to prance around, and play with my other memories. That cage was really heavy to mentally carry, anyway.

You know what? I think I deserve a bubble bath for facing down this passage. With *Gingerbread Latte* bubbles, and soft candles. My own personal spa treatment.

Now Boarding

It's only been one month since I sought help.

That's utterly insane, to me. A strong part of me suddenly feels weary. It's like I'm waiting for fate's twist that's going to take this tiny bit of hope, and courage I've regained, and smash it as it's been doing for some time now. I don't want to be scared though. If this feeling is only temporary, I want to enjoy it while it's here.

It feels like it has been much, much longer than a month that has gotten me to this point. It was while I was battling with my alarm clock that I realized it feels that way, because it has been a long time. The change didn't start a month ago, or after meeting Linda for the first time in October. It's been happening for several months now.

From what I can tell, it started when I mustered up the courage to stand up against my mother's moods while still living under the same roof. It was an easy choice after that time that I had decided to walk away from one of her temper tantrums. She threw my things out onto the front lawn as retaliation. After she went to work, I had gathered my belongings, and stayed at my Uncle John's for 3 or 4 days.

Also, I'm not trying to make out my mother as some bad guy. Just like with Cam, I know how odd that seems considering my constant complaints. The fact is, she has a very logic based mind. She grasps for control as her own survival mechanism. It does get boarder-line toxic at times, but only when she's under extreme stress. She cares and worries about me, and so wanted me to be the same.

I, however, use laughter, and the arts to survive. I sink into my fantasy worlds, and come up with elaborate stories that I hope to one day share with others.

The point is, when someone that relies on their logic first lives under the same roof as someone who's instinct is to follow their heart... there are bound to be misunderstandings, frustrations, and arguments.

Most of the time, I sat quiet while she ranted and raved at me. Then, one day, I started speaking my mind. It clearly never helped the situation. But, for the first time in a while, I did something for me without tip-toeing around. I wasn't letting Mum's doubts and fears pile on top of my own.

That eventually led to the next change. The fighting was getting worse, because even though I didn't fully realize it then, it was finally my time to go out, make my own choices, and learn to cope with the consequences as an independent young woman. Boy, did I make several bad choices. Still, they were mine to make, and mine to contend with. No matter how much it frustrates my loved ones to see me hurting.

The way I see it now, though, is that the stained glass art I'm forging into would need to undergo pressure to become a panel instead of a molten blob. For the record, I have no idea how glass panels are made, so if that metaphor is inaccurate, please just go with it. Or I could just resort to the "diamond from coal" cliché.

I am a firm believer that everything happens for a reason. I moved out on my own when I was in the middle of saving for a cross country trip to try out an industry that was suggested to me by some psychic. What if I had stayed under Mum's roof until I had made the needed money to go?

For one thing, I would have still been under her watchful eye. It would have frustrated me to no end, but worse still, it would have meant I wasn't learning to make decisions for myself. I would have also still been working at the call centre. Heaven only knows how much more my mind would have fractured under that stress. Sure, I would have been delighted to finally reach my goal of $50 grand. I would have hurried off to Vancouver, and made all my mistakes, and self-discoveries there.

I think that would have broken the last of whatever the

call centre spat out that resembled me.

Instead, I moved out, and had to learn how to take care of myself. I'm still terrible at that, but it's a work in progress.

At least, I'm not eating instant noodles every night.

I have two adorable little furballs that are my responsibility to care for. Which, they honestly take care of me too. Sometimes it's just nice to curl up with a rumbling purr in my ear, and a fuzzy back against my cheek. They keep me balanced.

I have had to deal with money troubles. It really put into perspective that I needed to figure out what to do. After I had left the call centre, I had $12,000 to survive off of. How badly did I want to pursue being a writer? Should I tuck it away to be a hobby only, or see how far I can get?

I learned the answer is I have the means and gift to be able to go all the way. It's just the courage I am lacking.

I chose to come back to school, even after dropping out of college once before. I did it as a plan to survive. I didn't want to be another welfare dependant. Plus, I wasn't even surviving that way. $681/month is not a lot when your rent is $637.50. Still, school was another choice.

Being an RPN was not for me, but I had the choice of any program, and any school across Ontario. I didn't have to limit myself to staying in Chatham anymore. I was free to go out there, and try new places. I was excited, but terrified. I had not said anything to my mother about applying to school until I was already doing so. Even after, it took another month or so before I admitted I had applied to a fine arts course.

I had applied to four different schools.

Niagara, Humber, Seneca, and Fanshawe. Niagara had been my first choice. Guess which one had been my last. The only reason I had bothered with Fanshawe was because I figured it might not be as competitive to get into as those from the bigger cities. It also helped that it was the closest arts related school to Chatham.

When I had applied shortly before the deadline in May, I was informed that I may be placed on a waiting list for Niagara.

Humber had been the first to get back to me with plenty of enthusiasm. They had even sent a little pin inside a golden ticket that read, "Humber student". Seneca and Fanshawe were fast to follow. I figured that if I couldn't go to Niagara, I wanted to go to Humber since they had got back to me first.

Except... call it fate, intuition, or divine intervention, I suddenly started to get anxious about living in Toronto. I'm not built for big cities. It's been taking a lot of adjusting just to settle into London. I'm still finding it very difficult to truly relax. I get close, though, when I'm in the art studio. I let my fear get the better of me, and accepted Fanshawe. The day after, the letter congratulating me to Niagara arrived in my mail. I could have changed, but I figured this was how it's supposed to be.

I don't regret it. This *is* where I am meant to be, right now. Close enough to my loved ones to easily hop a train to see them, or they take a drive to see me. Far enough for me to continue to learn and grow as my own self. The staff are amazing, and my classmates are perfect.

Being in the studios with paints, pencils, and fellow artist was like coming home. When I first got into sculpture, I was happy. I was in there every night for a week just trying new techniques with plaster. Seeing what worked and what didn't. I had never used it before, but I'd like to think that all five sculpts from project one had been a success.

It clicked: I am a sculptor. I mean, I knew for some time I liked to mess around with wet clay, but there's a difference between knowing you like to sculpt, and identifying yourself as a sculptor. Granted, I'm a stubborn fool, so I really only started to identify myself as such over the last week.

Now, I think of the painting I did for the self-portrait. I

made it look like a stain glass, which meant separating my face, and hair into their own parts. If I'm stain glass, then sculptor is one of those parts.

What I was feeling at the beginning was new, and overwhelming. It made lasting the full week of classes exhausting. Then, I would miss one. Then another. Any college student will tell you what a bad idea that is. Two missed classes meant a whole project behind. Suddenly, that little happy bubble popped around me. I panicked.

I'm sure I've said it many times in these passages, but I honestly believed I was going to fail.

I mean, that all sounds like a load of crap now. The thing is, I was already well into my transition. I couldn't go back, but I didn't know how to go forward. Against every instinct that told me otherwise, I sought help, and met Linda. She understood, and has been the master mind that connected me to the team of people that have been continually provoking me (intentionally and not) to wonder: What do I hope to achieve? Not just during and after school, but within my own centre.

Who am I?

When I jumped into writing this a month ago, a part of me was dying. The part that was broken beyond repair, and needed to be thrown away. It told me I was a coward, like my father. I was never going to amount to anything. Just a dreamer, and a slob, and a number of cruel things. It made me needlessly angry with people over petty things.

Really, Mum may have ditched my actual birthday for a concert, but she did realize how much it had hurt me. She couldn't stay and camp with me, but she had kept her word, and came out in time for campfire every night with goodies galore. I didn't just get to spend two hours with her over dinner on the 19th. I got to spend 3 or 4 hours with her over the course of three different evenings. I am so grateful for the times she uses those spare moments to be around me and Cam.

Also, so what if my sister likes to start fights with me

around her birthday? I fight back, and then she becomes legitimately upset for the day. If that's the pattern she wants, that's her prerogative. I'm sure I'll be pissed off if/when she does it again, but I still love her either way.

Which is why I remember now, what my second piece is: I'm forgiving.

I mean, it comes with it's pros and cons. A lot of cons when dealing with manipulative people.

Which is part three: I have trust issues.

Hey, not everything is all bright and cheery. The glass parts have to be held in place by cold metal bars, don't they?

I've been slighted enough times to spot a con artist a mile away. Unfortunately, it also makes me uncertain about whether someone's kindness is genuine, or backed by pity or selfish reasons. My classmates are a perfect example. During my October breakdown, any time I went to the class, I felt like I was a burden. I felt like a faker, and I had convinced myself that they all knew it. I was an outsider, in my mind's interpretation.

Yet, I've been met with understand from all of them. Plenty I want to call "friends", but instinct is telling me not to jump in, and be all clingy. No one likes a clingy person.

The fifth piece is that I'm a fighter. Actually, more accurately, I'm a survivor. In many ways, I am a bloody-coward, and in others, I'm the bravest bitch you could ever hope to have your back. I've had my fair share of shit storms. I know there are those that have had it better than me, and others that have had it far worse. It's not about who has a bigger pile to get through, though.

Despite the daunting task before me, I get out of bed with a shovel in hand. Heck, there are days the fucking thing is missing, and I have to use my bare hands to dig through this metaphorical crap. I'm still getting up, and getting through it. Sometimes there's a mud slide, and I need help getting free before I suffocate, but I'm still here. I'm still trying.

"I know I've got a chance. I just have to keep trying."

Six is still a new one for me. It's admitting that I'm not alright upstairs. For as much as I pride myself on my mind, there are parts that need healing. And that's okay. It's just mental health challenges. Not a disability. As I've just stated above, I'm not letting that shit weigh me down anymore. I'm going to be depressed. I'm going to loose my way, and anxiously worry about what to do next. I can't change that about who I am, but I have a team of people that are ready to teach me how to manage it. Professors that are willing to be patient with me, and classmates who understand.

I know Mum has issues about admitting I have these challenges. No parent wants to believe their child is hurting inside. Especially after all she did to make sure I grew up to be a bright, and independent woman. We're just going to have to work through it with time.

Finally, I saved the largest piece for last. Lucky number 7: I am kind.

Kind is such a broad word when you really think about it. It describes being friendly, polite, caring... a bunch of other examples my 2:30 am brain can't put together at this moment.

If this journal has shown me anything, it's reminded me of the common element that made me happiest: bringing joy to others. Entertaining them so that, for a moment, they don't have to worry about the shit pile they have to shovel through that day. If I can do that for the rest of my life, I will.

I want to jump-scare smirks, and nervous giggles in a haunted dungeon.

I want to dress up, and inspire a world of make-believe with some quick jokes, and a fake accent.

I want to see little eyes light up when they see the picture freshly painted on their face.

I want to tell jokes, and just be a goof-ball until sides are sore.

I want to spend hours listening to seniors and elders reminisce about things from before I was born. And learn the lessons hidden in their stories.

I want to build a theme park for people, and families to relax and play.

I want to tell stories. I don't care if it's through written word, or the silver screen.

If, only for the span of a blink, or the rest of my years, I can use my creative gift to bring people joy...

I would be the happiest, and most blessed woman alive.

Which leads me to my meeting today with a gentleman named Derek. When he asked me what I hoped to achieve, I told him I wanted to write, make movies, and sculpt. He spent the hour listening to me talk about my passions, and provided me with words of encouragement.

"It sounds like you have so many gifts to use. I feel honoured that I get to know you now."

I huffed a laugh at that.

"No, really. I believe there will be a day I will say to someone, 'I got to sit here with her'."

We spoke a little more into my writing. Then I mentioned how I had been writing for fourteen years. Out came the usual question about if I had published.

"No, but I own my own independent publishing unit," the practice line tumbles out.

Even if I have done nothing with my business, as of yet, it is still a successful step towards being a published writer, instead of just a hobbyist.

He presses on, "But you have manuscripts then..."

"Yeah, but they're not finished," I shrug. I'm just glad he didn't ask the "what's your book about" question.

"Why not?"

"Because I keep getting to a certain point, and then get a better idea. Then I end up going back, and rewriting the whole thing. Sometimes I just try to tweak something small, and end up having to rewrite the whole thing."

"What if you didn't go back to change things?"

I inwardly cringe. Last year, while I was giving writing my all, I knew another author named Cassie. Unlike me, she has actually completed her manuscripts, and published. She's the one that opened my eyes to the world of Indie writing and publishing. Cassie was even proof editing one of my partcilly done manuscripts for me. We talked a lot about both of our works. I ended up getting the farthest I had in a long time for book one, thanks to her help.

When I had told Cassie my issue, she warned me to stop.

"You're book is never going to be as perfect as you're trying to make it, but that doesn't mean it isn't good. You have to accept what you have made, and publish, or your never going to get past the first draft."

That was paraphrasing, by the way. I don't feel like hunting through my email history to get the exact wording at this moment, but, trust me when I say, she wrote it out so much more profound that I just did.

We haven't really interacted over the last year. She was busy doing the sequel to her book, and starting in on a miniseries. Meanwhile, I was too ashamed to admit I had started another re-write. After how much she has help me, I feel like I would be insulting her judgement.

"I don't know," I look away from Derek. "I just... start to feel unsure, and come up with a better idea."

"So you would say that you get anxious when you start getting closer to the end." I wasn't really sure if he was asking or stating that point.

I gave a small nod, "I guess."

"Is it because you are worried about what others will

think once you are published?"

Fucking nail on the head with that one. I loath to admit it, but, yes, I keep changing it because I want it to be able to be enjoyed by as many readers as possible. Anything I write, even this journal (which I'm starting to consider making available to a real audience instead of my imaginary one), makes me anxious about what readers will think.

Funny enough, for my original stuff it's the opinions of critics that scares me. For this journal, I fear my family were it to fall into their hands. it's worry about how my family will react.

I told Derek as much. His response was actually fairly decent.

"It's not their lives, though. Loved ones don't read something like that to understand. They are looking for something to criticize. One day, they will understand. But you have to go where your passion takes you. It's like a train. You're finally at the correct station. Now you just have to be brave enough to decide to get on. Don't just stand there, holding up your ticket, and let the train pass you by. Don't waste these gifts... your passion that you have."

Honestly, my first thought was the scene from the last Harry Potter movie (Because I'm the kind of fan that loves both the books and movies). The one where Harry is talking to Dumbledore in the between:

"We're at King's Cross, you say? I think if you so desired, you'd be able to board a train."

"And where would it take me?"

"On."

I feel the same could be said about what to do with my own train that Derek was talking about. He's right, I am finally at the station I need to be at. I can't just stand here like an idiot while my new life rolls away. After all, there's no way I want to go back to my self-loathing, self-pitying state that I was at only a few short weeks ago. I've come too far.

So...

Hold that train. I'm getting on.

Christmas Lights

I had stepped away from the journal for a while in order to focus on school and my personal writing projects. Surprisingly, I've apparently started a dependance on this journal. I think it's just nice to get my thoughts out there, instead of jumbled up inside my head.

Today is Tuesday, and I'm supposed to be at the school handing in the last of my projects. Except, they are not all finished. I'm waiting until 4 pm to go to the school, complete them, and then send the pictures to my professors. I plan to use the snow as an excuse for not meeting with the department coordinator, Gary, to hand things in. It's not like I had arranged a time with him, anyway.

I had been awake due to restlessness last night. Knowing that I was supposed to go today after being given a second chance, and then not having all of it finished made me want to run to the school to finish them. Except walking at 3 am in a city is dangerous enough without factoring in snow and ice.

London was hit with about a foot of snow. Of course, I was ecstatic. I actually had to take a walk in it, just to feel the crunch under my boots, and the cool against my cheeks. It was not as cold as you would have expected a snow storm to be. It lacked the bitter, biting chill that some of the fall days had had.

Unfortunately, I think my strolling in a winter wonderland has me coming down with a cold. Completely worth it, so long as it stays as sniffles for Christmas.

Look at that, the perfect transition.

You know, at one time it was part of a tradition for Mum to spend a day with Cam and I just decorating. We would go wild with it too. Two Christmas trees, both full of ornaments and topped with an angel. There would be red and gold garland hanging from the ceiling. At the centre of the garland waves was a beautiful folding star. The outside of the house was much simpler with lights hanging from the eavestrough, and wrapped around the trees.

We had one of those free-standing, pre-lit reindeer. For whatever reason, ours never wanted to stay upright. It never mattered where we put him in the front yard. After a while, Mum didn't want to put him out at all, but I still did every year. Besides, it started to become a running joke about how long it would take before Jack Frost killed Rudolph, again.

Funny thing is, the neighbour across the street had one that was fine. Of course, their one reindeer has steadily started growing into a herd. The last time I visited Chatham, Mum and I laughed to see he had about eight or nine strewn across the front yard.

There was also another neighbour from three doors over, and across the street, who really outdoes themselves with lights. I've seen her out in her yard, and it usually takes about a day to set up. In fact, I think last year took her a second day. It's not that big of a front yard, but that just makes it look like something you would expect from a department store window. Candy canes, blow-up snowmen, and even a little train. You could stand there for an hour just taking the sight in.

One year, Mum had come to pick Cam and I up from somewhere, and told us she had a surprise for us. My jaw dropped as the front of our house was done up with a million different lights. It still wasn't the mayhem from down the street, but it was definitely a lot more than we usually put up. Mum had set it up without us knowing.

"What do you think?" You could hear the giddiness in Mum's voice.

Before I could say anything, my sister blurted out, "That's it?"

Two little words was all it took to destroy Mum's hard work, and my Christmas-y joy. I spent a good hour trying to give Mum as many compliments about it as I could. I was trying to over compensate for my sister's lack of enthusiasm about the surprise. The damage was done, though, and Mum went back to doing only simple lights outside.

As we got older, Mum couldn't be as bothered to dazzle the house as much as before. I know there was also a period where, during my teenaged years, I didn't want to spend hours cleaning, decorating, and then taking it down in a handful of weeks. It was too much effort. Eventually, we stuck to one tree, and our lazy reindeer. Sometimes Mum would help, but, mostly, she would order Cam and I to do it.

When I started working at the call centre, I began to return to that decorative vibe my mother once had. When Christmas came around, I went all out with dollar store lights, plush snowmen, false mini-trees, and garland and snowflakes galore.

Plus, being one that can never sit still, I spent a lot of time folding origami. I had learned how to make a paper crane when I was thirteen. Ever since, I would cut up entire pages into little squares, colour them, and then fold them. I eventually figured out how to fold them a certain way to have patterned wings with solid coloured bodies. I'm sure I still have the box of my favourites that I had kept tucked away somewhere around here.

Cranes are not the only thing I make anymore. I make 3D stars, butterflies, and frogs from memory too. My favourite though was taught to me by a nice woman at the call centre, but only after I made a crane in front of her.

What did she teach me? A dragon.

Once I had learned the dragon, and taught her the frog, the two of us had started this creative friendship. Any time one of us learned something new, we would teach the other. It's been a long time since I learned how, but I could do a paper flower ball thanks to her. I have a small one made from gold foil around somewhere.

I used to also know how to make little present boxes. So,

by the time the 25th rolled around, my desk, and many of my friends' desks, were covered with origami present boxes. My favourite ones are currently hanging on strings from my tree - high enough for my cats not to reach.

    Yes, my apartment has been decorated since November 12th.

    The point is that I am very much one of those Christmas spirits. It's the one time of year that I am guaranteed a few hours with my mother and sister. The jokes as we exchange presents can be seen in our grins in every photo taken. Maybe it's the lights reflecting off the snow, or the quiet peace winter brings. I swear, for the entire season, the world just feels so much brighter.

    I really wish it could feel like this all the time.

All You Need is Love

    I am definitely feeling sentimental right now. I was just thinking about my loved ones. Especially those that I tend to have hiccups with.

    I think I'll start with my grandmother. Remembering the fall out with Nick made me think that she does have my back. It may not always seem like she cares because her attention is more on other members of my family, but she does in her own way. It's in how we joke with one another. By joke, I mean random insults being flung back and forth. It's in the times we play cards, or go fishing together. She showed she cared when I first moved out, and she not only helped me move, but also brought two boxes, and one of those big Walmart bags full of things I would need now that I was living on my own. There were times I needed a ride somewhere, and she came to get me. I know we fight a lot. It's hard not to when you're close to someone. Still, at the end of the day, I love my grandma. Sassy attitude, and all.

    Next is my Aunt Heather. I know I often feel like I'm just a burden to her. It's one of the reasons I have such a hard time randomly texting her to say hello. I feel like I'm just in her way. I also know that she doesn't think any of that. Even on her busiest days, I've been welcomed to her home. She's helped me take the steps I needed to find my own place to live when my mother wouldn't. She believes in me, and listens to me. She's protective of me, and cares, even when things are upside down in her own life. I try to show her the same amount of support that she shows me, but I don't think I could ever get close.

    That's why I love my Aunt Heather.

    Aunt Heather's son, Wilson. I know I don't talk about him much. He's a good kid. Sometimes I worry about him because of some of the friends he has. But I know he's got a good head on his shoulders, and is stronger inside than he knows.

I love that kid.

My Uncle John, Aunt Sandra, and the kids, Sonia and Dean. I miss them. I miss them all so much. Uncle John is an amazing artist, and very much a gamer. You can tell Sonia loves and is trying to be like her daddy. As for Sandra, I was wary of her when she first started dating my Uncle. She quickly became part of the family, however. I miss our girl talks. She one of few people in my family who really seems to get some of the difficulties I face. Then there's Dean. What a wild-fire. He's going to be a heart break when he's older.

I love each of them, and miss them.

My sister, Camilla. She frustrates me about as many times as I frustrate her. We fight, and bicker, and there have been times we went months without talking. Yet, I wouldn't trade her for the world. When I feel at my worst, I get in contact with her. When I find a silly video, or just want to talk about random shenanigans, it's her that I want to share with. She makes me laugh. I love the days we can just sit together, and laugh about the sarcastic assholes that we are. I know she is always there for me. Just like how I'm always keeping an eye out on her.

She's my absolute best friend. For all we piss each other off, I love her just the way she is.

Finally, the most complicated for last, my Mum. I have to remember that I'm not a disappointment to her. I don't have to keep striving to earn her love. She already loves me the way I am. No, she doesn't care about my writing, but not everyone will. To me, it feels like she's not accepting me, then, but that's not it. I have to remember that there is a difference between supporting a particular piece of work, and supporting me. She's there for me as an artist. I can send her pictures of my projects, and she celebrates with me.

She loves me enough that, even if I wasn't planned, she kept me and raised me. Even when she worked long hours, she made time for us. Even if she had to work her ass off, she made sure we had everything we could ever want and need. I don't get to see her a lot, and she may not call me everyday, but she still checks in on me when she can.

She's fiercely protective of me... even if it means trying to save me from myself. She worries about me, especially when I get some ambitious idea in my head. She was there for me through my crushes. I mean, seriously, she snuck a picture of my Grade 8 crush during our graduation! I found it during one of the many times I was going through family pictures.

She may have her own skeletons to contend with. There's a lot of factors that can strain our relationship, from either side. Still, I have to remember that she does love me. As both her daughter, *and* as myself as an individual. She raised me into who I am, and I will always be grateful for that.

I love my mum. I hope she knows, and never has reason to doubt that.

I know they care about me as much as I care about them. They are my inspiration to keep getting up each morning. I'm not alone in this world. I can do so much because of them.

I need to remember that, especially the next time I'm in the middle of one of my episodes. I am me, and I have people that love me for it.

Grumbling

It's nearly 2:30 AM. I'm much too tired to be awake at this hour. Doesn't help that I'm hungry, as well, but I dare not sneak downstairs for food. One, the dogs will bark and wake Mum. Two, I feel like a guest, not at home, so I feel the need to ask to get food, or an extra blanket. I feel like Mum would be miffed if I made myself too comfortable.

That's probably an anxiety related paranoia kicking in.

As you can tell, I am, currently, at my mother's house. In my old bedroom, to be exact. I'm visiting until Saturday, the 17th, then I'm going home until Christmas. It's Thursday, now, considering it's past midnight. I know Mum intends to have me up before 7 to go battle gyms in the Pokemon Go app. She's a little obsessed.

That being said, none of that is why I am writing tonight when I'm quiet comfortable enough to sleep. Not more than my own bed, sadly, but it's comfortable as in a peaceful sort of thing. I think it's the fact that Mum hasn't changed the wallpaper from the wild cat wonder it's been since I was 10. That, and it's still the same furniture, and I did sleep in this room for thirteen years. This was the first room I had ever had that was mine, alone.

Cam and I had shared our bed while growing up. When we moved in with Nicholas, in his two bedroom home, we had to share a bed since the tiny second bedroom could only fit one bunk-bed with it's dressers. Cody was a bed wetter for some time, so he and James got the bottom bunk. Better to have two piss covered children, than to let it drip through the top bunk, and have all four of us a mess.

I always felt bad for James for having to be put through that. I mean, my sister was a terrible bed hog, and only made things worse with a dozen large stuffies. At least, she was not a bed wetter.

That also meant that the mattress could not be slept on during the other days of the week when the boys were not there. I suppose it didn't bother me except when I would have to, nightly, push my sister away from me so that I actually could stretch out.

Once I had my own space, however, it was mine, and I hated people invading it. Cam was the same way.

The difference was, I respected my sister's space, while she was constantly in my room. A lot of times, without me there so that she could just take what she wanted.

I hated lending things to her. I once used my Christmas money to get myself a portable DVD player. At first, I was reluctant to let her use it, but Mum told me that I had to, or it would be taken away. Cam ended up having it more often than I did, and, Heaven forbid, I asked for it back. It was eventually swallowed up by the mess of her room. It was recovered many years later, buried and broken.

Honestly, that annoys me still that I budgeted my Christmas money to buy myself something nice, and my sister takes it while she used her own Christmas cash on other things. Thing is, I had known she had my portable DVD player, so it didn't surprise me when we found it during her bedroom clean out. I had not, however, ever lent her my paint brushes.

I can't remember if it was from my summer job at Dairy Queen, or by using birthday money, but the result was that I had bought a cheap set of 24 brushes.

When I spent my seven months in Brazil, I came home to my bedroom being temporarily used by one of Mum's work friends. The friend was in a bad situation, and so had needed a place to stay until she could get things figured out. They had been aiming to get her settled before I was meant to get home, but my three month early return had meant my room was still occupied by someone else. I tried to not show my possessiveness, and didn't mind using the much larger bed in the basement-basement.

What I had not know is that they had cleared out some of my drawers of things (including my craft drawer) to make room for clothing. I had searched high and low for my brushes, once I had my room back. Hardly a year later, I finally found them. Again, in my sister's room, buried under junk, and snapped from being repeatedly stepped on to get to her bed.

So much for, "I don't know where your brushes are."

Great, I'm being bitter tonight. It honestly has not been one of my strong days today. It's not that there was anything particularly wrong with today. In fact, quiet the opposite. It just feels off. These back and forth swings makes me wonder if maybe I should be medicated. Suppose that's a question for another day.

Don't Touch the Switch

It's nearly 1 am on the 17th of December. In twelve hours, Mum and I will be driving for some town that's on the way to London. That's where her cousin, my Aunt Yolanda, lives. We're celebrating family Christmas there, and then Mum is taking me home.

Funny, when I'm in London, I think of Chatham as home, but when I'm in Chatham, it's the other way around.

I think I forget how busy my family is. They always want to be on the go with something, and I'm used to being laid back, and enjoying the quiet. Since Mum had to work an afternoon shift, I got the chance to breathe for a few hours.

Cam had wanted to hang out almost instantly after Mum left. I had said "sure" at first, but then I text her back to decline. She still came over, insisting that I will be going with her.

I held my ground, and said, "no thank you." It clearly annoyed her, but I needed that time.

Plus, I know all she wanted was to dye my hair. I don't understand her obsession with it. I actually am quiet fond of the natural colour. At least, when my hair is freshly cleaned. She, however, likes making my hair various shades of deep red. She thinks gingers are awesome, and my light, freckled skin plus bright green eyes are already really close. Still, I often let her just because it's bonding time, and it makes her happy. Plus, some times, it's nice to go a different look for a bit.

This time, though, I really did not want to. I managed to avoid it while visiting yesterday, which is why she was so persistent about doing it today. She had bought the dye while her, Grandma, and I were out and about. Apparently, she was mixing it up this time, because she chose blonde.

Still, I got my quiet time. First I caught up on sleep. Then

I took the time to read through some of my earlier passage. It was really tempting to edit it, but I managed to only correct typos. It was interesting to see the beginning changes in myself.

The part about Joy telling me to exercise more reminded me I should. Contrary to what my size might indicate, I actually really like exercise. Once I get myself to get going, anyway.

Thing is, I can't just hop on a treadmill, and go for hours. Anything that gives me too much time to think can be dangerous. It's why, despite preferring slow and quiet life style, I need to be around a small group of friendly people, or out in nature. It's much easier to ground myself.

Still, Dr Adams was riding my ass at our last meeting (on Monday) about exercising more. She said I am making progress with my depression, and thinks my lifestyle choices are holding me back from going further.

Truth is, my depression isn't better. It's just been easier to ignore. It's like I told Linda that one time:

"I have a switch. So long as things are good, the switch remains off. As soon as I start to panic about any little thing, the switch is flipped, and I sink into my full depression."

I know this about myself. That's just the way it has always been. The reason Dr Adams thinks I'm improving is because she had first met me while school stress had flipped my switch. Right now, the switch is being left alone.

My anxiety is still being a hassle. I'm worried that I didn't make the grade to continue next semester. Heck, I'm worried about my Mum seeing my apartment because I know she's going to make negative comments.

I hate when she does that, by the way. I know what things are a mess, where. The fact it's a mess really annoys me, but I have to scrounge up some energy to do anything about it. Not to mention, she will be on me about the things not done, that she will completely overlook what is done. Case in point, before she picked me up on Wednesday, I had scrubbed my shower, toilet, and bathroom sink. All of which is going to escape her notice, even though she is probably going to need to use my bathroom.

So, yeah, anxiety is there, but nothing major is setting me off. Thus, I'm as emotionally balanced as I can hope to be. We'll see what tomorrow holds, though. Mum is going to stress over getting everything ready for the Christmas party, and being there on time when there is fresh snow as of tonight. It's going to set her on a negative spin, which usually means she going to get moody, and controlling.

Chances are, she's going to say something that's going to hit my switch. Which is why I really should be in bed right now.

Christmas with the Sporidnenyy

I called it. As expected, Mum stressed, and we clashed. Now I'm awake at 12:30 AM, not really sure what to do with myself.

So, here I am; writing to imaginary readers, again.

Okay, my grandmother's side of the family had Christmas today. This included Grandma's brother, his two daughters, the significant other of said daughters, five of his grandchildren, and his one great-granddaughter. We call Grandma's brother, Uncle Fred. It was probably because he was my mother's uncle, and we didn't know what else you're supposed to call the uncle of your parent. Honestly, I'm still not sure. I assume he's my great-uncle, or something along those lines.

This year, we had the extended family Christmas (on grandma's side) at my Aunt Yolanda's house. She's the older of Uncle Fred's daughters, and mother to my cousins, Trevor, Erin, and Ian.

Oh right, Erin's boyfriend was here too. I'm sure you can tell it was a full house. At the same time, it wasn't really. Aunt Yolanda has a huge, 6 bedroom home in Delaware. She used to live in something even bigger than that, but downsized a few years back. Honestly, walking through her house, I smirk thinking about the fact I would build Sims 3 houses very similar in space and design. If that isn't a sign I play too much, I don't know what is.

Mum was fussing already today about little things she needed to get done. The tree needed to be put up, because she doesn't like doing it alone, yet blames it 'needing' to be up on Cam and I. There were things to pack, and gifts to wrap. You could tell it was bothering her, because she was repeating a list of everything that still need to be done. The more stressed she visibly got, the more on edge it made me. I'm sure if I had done anything wrong, including simply standing too close, she would have started yelling and berating me.

She started to talk about calling in for the one hour lunch feed to give herself more time. While I was under the tree, trying to get the stand straight, she was on about her fourth or fifth time explaining why she should call in. I knew she was not saying it for my sake.

I peeked up at her, and, as reassuringly as I could, I said, "Mum, you don't have to worry about explaining to me. If you want to call in, then I think you should. Clearly your, um, you know... getting a little stressed."

By the end of it, I was suddenly terrified that the last part of what I said would anger her instead of help.

She did, a little, but was more taken back from what I could tell, "Well... yeah. I mean, I have..." And then she started in on her list, again.

She got about half-way through, and I risked interrupting, "Then why don't you call?"

"I'm going to," she countered. "I'm just waiting a couple minutes so that..." she rattled off a reason. By then, I had returned to my work under the tree.

I am happy to say that she was much calmer. Especially after she did call in, and wasn't as frazzled. I did what I could to help where I could, even if it just meant staying out of her way. She was still on my ass, though, so I secretly flipped her off at one point to make myself feel better. That was over the fact I did not having my laundry done.

See, she had been nice enough to tell me I could bring all of my laundry (bedding included) to be washed for free. I had jumped at the offer, but had not got all of it finished by the time she was ready to leave. Mostly because she doesn't want the washer running during certain hours, and needed it for her own things in between.

That may seem unrelevant to the story, but trust me. It is.

At last, I was all too happy to be on the road. I really like this side of my family. They are busy, and so loud they make my sister and I seem soft spoken. Miraculously, the two of us were having a hard time being heard most of the night.

Noise aside, they are happy, and affectionate people. I always feel a little awkward around my extended family, because I don't know them well enough to know what they like, and what topics to keep away from.

The Sporidnenyy family, though, are so jolly and friendly, it's easy to tell how we are related. I don't worry so much about if I'm acting too much like a Burns, because there is a large chunk of my mother's family that is the same way. I really could be taking after either side.

One thing I knew they were going to love was the game, *Cards Against Humanity*. Last year I had brought *Apples to Apples*, and somehow we had turned it into a hilarious, dirty game. I knew *Card Against Humanity* would exaggerate that. My Uncle John (who doesn't go to these functions because Sandra's anxiety won't let them go near the bustling bunch) had bought the game some time ago. We only got to play it once because Sonia was listening in a little too closely, and had started saying "dirty butt hole" at school.

Thankfully, he let me borrow it. I was beyond excited to get to the party and play. I said as much to Mum, with a grin that was making my cheeks sore.

"Well, we might not even get time to play it," Mum stated.

I had to clamp my jaw in order to not make a comment about her having something against me being excited. I ended up silent for ten minutes while Mum started talking about casual stuff. Eventually we did start to chat, and things lightened up some. An hour later, and we made it. Which lead to the next hiccup of the night.

As I was gathering things to take inside, I made sure to grab my little jar of Spicy Red Pepper Jelly. I tucked it into my coat pocket, which Mum saw.

"Why are you putting that in your pocket?" She snapped.

I didn't know how to answer. I had been telling her since I brought it on Wednesday that I wanted the family to try it. Why was she getting mad at me for bringing it in like I had intended?

When I didn't answer, she got more snippy, "You're going to forget it."

True, I had forgotten it in Mum's fridge since she was rushing me out the door. I figured it was meant to be an appetizer spread, though, and, once dinner started, I could just put it away in my pocket so that I wouldn't forget it. Once again, however, I could not convey this to my mother.

She huffed in aggravation, "Whatever." Then stormed off to inside, leaving me to carry the bin with the gifts and food inside. She didn't even help with the front door. Instead, she went to greet her cousins as if she hadn't just started to loose her cool with me over a jam jar.

Really, the whole thing made me feel like I was 12 again, not 25.

The rest of the night went fantastic. Grandma loved the jam, as I knew she would. Cam, and Aunt Tammy (Yolanda's sister) tried it too, and liked it. I came to learn it's also great on pumpernickel bread. We had a large dinner that gave me time to sit and chat with my cousin, Ian.

The gift exchange was fun, as well. You see, we don't buy gifts for one another. There is just too many of us, and keeping track of who wants what is a pain. Instead, we play that game where you pick a number from a hat, and take turns either stealing, or grabbing an unwrapped gift from the pile. My first gift I picked was a wine glass with "Owl love you for always". Of course there was a little owl on it. Mum had wanted it.

Funny, seeing as I made that painting for her last year that was almost the exact same thing. Whatever.

After Trevor stole Aunt Yolanda's deep-frier, she stole my

wine glass. I decided to pick a fresh gift, hoping to get the $25 cash I knew was hidden in there somewhere.

Didn't find it, but I did get a nice new throw blanket and some chocolates. No one stole it from me.

Also, as it so happened, even with our limited time, we were still able to play two other games. One being *Cards Against Humanity*. Which Grandma won, of course. That's the thing about playing any sort of card game with her; she always draws the best cards. It's frustrating, yet fun because then it's your skill against her luck. Today, luck won.

The other game was an impromptu search game started by Aunt Tammy. Aunt Yolanda does this challenge with her children. They have until Christmas to find a tiny ornament in the tree in exchange for $20. Anyone that knocks over the tree, or breaks one of the other ornaments is instantly disqualified for this year, and next.

Tammy decided she was going to be the one to find it. Cam, Erin, and I joined her. Mum and Grandma would shout out suggested spots for us.

The ornament in question is a plastic pickle about the size and thickness of the pinky finger's top knuckle. The damn thing happens to also be the exact shade of green as the tree. After years of doing this, and the fact the tree was about 7 feet tall, Aunt Yolanda has become a master at hiding it.

Needless to say, despite several of us searching, no one found it.

The night was winding down, which lead to what truly turned things sour. On the way up to Delaware, Mum had made it clear she did not want to stay too late because there was supposed to be bad weather coming. During the car ride, she mentioned that if it turns out to be too bad, she'll just take me with her back to her place.

She left out the part about not taking me home until Monday afternoon.

So, it's time to head home, and there's word that the roads are a little slick. Mum jumps at the fact she's taking me back to her place, and THEN mentions she won't be able to bring me home tomorrow.

Another overnight at my mother's wasn't going to hurt.

Another two days was going to cause me to go into an emotional breakdown. Especially since, with Christmas getting closer, she's getting more stressed. That makes being under the same roof as her more toxic. I had already just spent three days walking on egg shells.

I had even gone hungry for the majority of the time I was there, because I didn't want her pissed at me for either a) cooking something she didn't want me to make and/or b) dirtying her dishes. It may sound like unfounded reasons to starve one's self, but these are legitimate things I have been scolded for multiple times (even while living with her).

Plus, I knew that the longer I stayed, the more she would expect me to do for her. I don't mind helping since she has a bad back, but there's a difference between asking, and expecting something to be done.

Finally, there was the matter of my cats. I had given them enough food to last them until I got home tonight. It's one thing for me to go hungry for a couple hours, but it's another matter for them to be left to starve for two days.

Mum seemed to predict the last train of thought because she pressed, "your cats will be fine."

My mind spun in search of another answer. I asked Erin if she was going to London, since I knew she lived there, but she was staying at her mom's for the night. Aunt Yolanda said she could take me in the morning.

It was better than Monday, but I still wanted to go home tonight. "I just don't know about all of my stuff..."

I could also feel Mum growing annoyed behind me. "Look, I don't want to drive a half an hour the other way, and then have to drive all the way back to Chatham," she growled. It was that tone that I knew meant I had no choice in the matter, and had better stop stalling.

I knew that it was not an unreasonable desire, but neither was my want to go home. I tried to think of another alternative to meet middle ground, but Mum had enough.

"Fine! I'll just fucking put my life in danger!" She aggressively pulled on her boots, and stormed out the door.

I could feel my stress level rising as I grabbed the bin, and followed Mum out to the van. I told myself it was going to be okay. Yeah, I would have to put up with her bitching at me for the next half-hour, and then getting the silent treatment for the next week while she mouths off about me to anyone that would listen behind my back. But at least I was going home.

Or so I thought.

As soon as we were both seated in the van, she really started in on me. "I don't see why you can't just come back to my place. I'm working until one on Monday, and can take you home straight after. Your cats will be fine until then."

"No they won't," I snip. "They'll already be out of food by today."

"Then why don't you spend the night at Yolanda's, and she can take you home in the morning, and I'll bring you your things later."

"I didn't realize that was an option," I argued, thinking she meant she would bring my things on Monday. "I'll grab my over-night bag, and go ask."

"Take the cooler with you, and ask if you can put it into her fridge, or something," she countered. I gathered both, and as I closed the sliding back door, Mum added, "Looks like I get to carry your shit around in my van for the next week!"

I knew what she was doing. She was trying to get me to change my mind, just so I would have my things. Otherwise, I'm to go without for a week.

I chose my sanity, and being out from under her control. Tomorrow I get to go home without any bedding, and only the clothing in my bag to wear for the next week. Oh, and most of the food including my bowl of left overs, the Ukrainian noddles Grandma had made just for me, and my gift, were all in her van too.

Merry Fucking Christmas.

Cam and our grandparents were leaving at the same time, so they got a front row view of Mum's mini-fit. When I had come from the van carrying my bag, and the small cooler, Cam asked if I needed help. The look on her face meant she had something to say, but didn't want it said in front of our grandparents, or within Mum's earshot.

Turns out, Cam was pissed. Probably more angry than Mum had been moments before.

"Yeah, Erin had asked if everything was okay after you guys left. I looked at her and told her that was normal." Her pace was sped up by heated temper. I, being in a subdued mood, was slowed, and so a little bit behind her when she proceeded to open the front door, and go up to Yolanda.

"My mother is being a bitch, so can Anita stay the night?"

Yolanda had been more than understand. When I apologized "for the episode", her response was, "What episode?" At first I thought she misunderstood what I was getting at, but, after I repeated myself, she smiled, and asked again, "*What* episode?"

Yolanda, and her boyfriend, Don, were super nice about setting me up in the spare room. Honestly, I was about ready to cry from the contrast of their kindness to my mother's wrath. I would have curled up, and secretly cried in the room, but Yolanda kept pointing out that they were watching a movie downstairs. It was obviously an invite. I figured it would have been rude to hide away when I was a guest.

We ended up watching *How the Grinch Stole Christmas*

(the live action version).

    Cam did text to check on me while watching the movie. I text back that I wasn't okay, but I would survive. I knew that Mum was going to talking shit about me, and give me the cold shoulder for the next week. At least, I am no where near her to actually have to put up with it. It's lucky I have other throw blankets, too, so I do have something to sleep with. In the end, Mum didn't get what she wanted.

    It turns out, she has already started her bullshit by calling Grandma, according to Camilla. She said that Grandma was giving Mum shit for treating me like that. I told her to tell Grandma, "thank you".

    That combined with my sister's support made things a lot better. Sometimes you just need the reminder, not just a self-assurance, but to actually witness it, that you are loved.

    Well, it seems my exhaustion is finally outdoing my restless anxiety. I'm going to sleep, and just hope for a better tomorrow.

You Do What You Can

The last two days have been odd.

To start, I'd like to be clear that, under extreme stress when already struggling with mental health, the body tends to react in various ways. I know a woman who says she went blind in one eye for 2 years. She said the Doctors could not find anything wrong with her, until eventually she was placed on anti-depressants. She claims that a week on the medication and she regained her vision. I have no idea if any of it was true or not, but it get's the point that a broken mind can do a lot of havoc on the body.

I have had moments where stress has done odd things to me as well. Mostly, I'm either lethargic and almost blacking out from sheer exhaustion (I actually made a hospital trip while at St Clair because of this one), or I'm vomiting to the point I'm painfully heaving bile.

Being jolted awake at 8 am on Sunday because I had apparently lost control of my bladder was a new one. I'm still mortified. I mean, it's one thing if I had been drinking. Thing is, I had not had a drop, *and* I was up only five hours prior to use the toilet. It just did, and I was woken from a dead sleep by it. I'm just glad instinct had roused me, and no one else was awake. Thankfully, it did not occur again this morning.

After cleaning myself up, I ended up going back to bed, and sleeping until almost noon. When I did get up, Aunt Yolanda was ready, and had me out the door to go home in under 10 minutes.

I was annoyed, because my cousins had helped themselves to my yogurt. I don't think they realize my fridge and freezer are scary low right now. I still have noodles, can goods, and a couple boxes of rice to last me the week. The leftovers that I had taken from dinner on Saturday ended up being left in my mother's van after our spat. They would have really come in handy. I don't have any money to spare towards groceries.

That aside, on a good note, I had two visitors yesterday. The first, and more surprising one, was my friend, Lynn. I had first met her when I joined one of the speciality divisions of the call centre we worked at. She's incredibly kind, and has a quick wit that always seems to catch me off guard. Of course, she's got several years more practice at sarcasm than me.

Apparently, one of the businesses she does (on top of still working at the call centre) had her driving to a city past London. Since she was in town around supper time, she had text me to ask if I wanted to get an early dinner. We met up at the Tim's down the street which was my suggestion, since I still had a Tim's card. It had been a gift from Mum some time ago.

I was more than happy to see Lynn, and hang out. Admittedly, I'm terrible at keeping in contact with people. I feel like I'm bothering them if I message too often. Especially if I message them first more times than they do in a month. I still consider them a friend, though. There are people I haven't spoken to in years, and if they called me up wanting to hang out, I'd be there.

Luckily, Lynn is the same way.

She's one of the few people I know that I can go some time without talking to, and it never changes our friendship.

Her company yesterday was at a perfect timing. I was in a poor frame of mind when she text. For one thing, there was the issue with my mother, and knowing that this is going to carry over to Christmas itself. For another, I had a dozen things to do before meeting with Gary the following day (which is now, today). I was, and still am, terrified that I will fail one of my classes. It's only going to take one to keep me from returning, and starting fresh in the winter semester.

Yeah. Here I had been given second, third, and even fourth chances. Yet my lazy, procrastinating ass couldn't get out of bed and just work on the five projects I had left. That's right, FIVE projects. I did, albeit messily and hurried, finish the two painting projects. I did the costume for my 2D and 3D media this morning before my meeting at noon.

Lynn's visit did help me find some courage to still go to the meeting. I brought in my sorry projects, and left them out to display on the table. I knew Gary was going to be in a meeting about final grading with all the other fine art teachers. He had called me earlier to tell me this so that we could make arrangements to bring in my projects.

When we had spoke, he made it sound like I didn't need to be there. With everything spread out, I hurry off to the Quiet Room. I didn't want to be there when Gary and my professors came in, and saw how terrible of a job I had done.

Unfortunately, as I was heading for the stairwell, I heard someone call out my name. I turned to look, and it was Gary. Both my Painting, and 2D/3D professors were with him.

"Do you got a minute?" he greeted cheerfully.

My stomach dropped. I swear my blood pressure sky-rockected. I meekly nodded, and followed back to the studio. I know there were a couple times he had turned to say something to me, but I can't remember what. I just continued to nod. I didn't want to risk panicking, and crying.

I did end up crying, though.

It wasn't anything anyone had said. They were actually really nice, even Gary. The last time I had talked to him, he had scolded me about not doing my work. I was rather surprised he was being so understanding. My painting professor didn't say much either. He just took pictures of the paintings and research work, and kept the topics to strictly classwork.

It was my own head whispering over and over, *"You're going to fail. You don't have this done for this class. You didn't do any of your portfolio work. How could you be so stupid? You should have had it done weeks ago. You've thrown away every chance these people have given you. Way to go. So, how are you going to pay your rent come February?*

As if your lazy ass can hold a job. If you can even get one in time. You're going to have to go back to Chatham, and tell everyone you're a failure."

A small voice of hope tried to counter it. Yes, I was missing the portfolio, but I had all of my painting projects in. That's 80% of my grade.

I may be missing one sculpture, and my portfolio, but I had been doing well in Sculpture. Three projects still counted for 60% of my grade weight. I knew 20% was almost perfect.

The one I was most worried about was 2D and 3D media. I knew the costume was one of the higher weighted projects, but I don't know if it would be enough to offset the marks to pass. I was almost certain that I was going to fail that one.

The cruel inner voice knew this, and using it against me.

My painting professor apparently needed another picture of my first project. I thought he had already had it, but, fortunately, I had it in my locker. It was while I was at my locker that Christine (2D/3D professor) came over to talk to me. I was already on the verge of tears, and she was trying to talk me through it.

I admitted where my thoughts were, and she kept saying, "It's okay. You've done what you could. I'm pretty sure everyone here already knows what's going on."

Trying to internally grasp onto those words while the voice in my head was screaming at me is what finally broke the flood gate. Just a crack, though. I was able to get myself in check, and cleaned up in under two minutes. During that, Christine took my project one painting from me to give to my painting professor on the other side of the wall of locker-cupboards.

When I came around, Christine was trying to be encouraging again. For the record, this is a woman that I found intimidating. There was a moment, though, while I was crying, that I could see on her face, and hear in her voice that she wasn't just being sympathetic. She's been through the fire too.

I couldn't look her directly in the eye, mostly because my vision was blurry. I can't say if I noticed it was still in her, or not. I came to learn that there's another type of forge survivor. One where the external facade was cool, like the steel formed ones, yet, internally, was an amazing stain-glass.

I wonder what I should call this type of survivor?

During our conversation, I realized I had one more opportunity. She was telling me that I just do what I can about getting a picture to her with me wearing the costume... which I just realized I completely forgot to do. Shit. I was to have it to her by midnight.

"Hey, since I'm already here at the school, maybe I can finish up project 6, too?" I tentatively asked.

Christine was more than happy to jump on board with the idea. I did get it done, too. It's simple, and definitely not worth a lot in marks, but, it's like she said.

"Even if it's just a 50, that's still 50% better than a 0."

With all the projects done in 2D and 3D media, as well as Painting, I may just scrap by. The only one I have left to worry about it Sculpture.

Since the grades mechanic will be down until 4 pm on the 21st -starting sometime tomorrow, the 20th- it's going to be a couple days until I know if I've passed or failed.

Oh, and I just remembered my second visitor last night was Nick. However. it was just a visit. No sex. He even started in on his game when it was time for bed. I made a joke, then turned over and went to sleep. That had clearly bothered him, from what I got from his text message later.

I sent him a message to thank him for being there for me when I was stressing out last night. He did make a couple jokes about having to take care of things himself. He also mentioned, near the end of the conversation, that he'd be willing to come over again to be a bed heater, since I still don't have my blankets from my Mum.

Which, for the record, I find it incredibly annoying. I already over heat in my sleep. I've had to resort to keeping the window open a crack at night, since my fan is currently broken (and I have no idea why). Plus, he's too fucking clingy. Maybe I'm just used to sleeping on my own, and moving as I please on a full Queen size.

I guess instinct from sharing a bed with my clingy sister when we were children is still there too. I don't know, and seeing as it's now 4 am, I don't really care.

I know it's only the one visit. Still, it's a small victory, so I'll take it.

Kidlets and Chijens

I have to say, I woke up in a fighting mood this morning. It might have something to do with Mum sending me a message yesterday:

"Why the hell did you unplug my damn couch?"

The simple answer is, I didn't.

Any other time, she would not have cared. Since she's angry with me, and no one is siding with her, she's looking for an outlet. Real fucking mature.

Seeing as I knew full well what she was doing, I didn't answer back. I did tell my sister that I don't want to come back to Chatham for Christmas if I have to deal with that. She got pretty pissed off about the way Mum is acting. We could not chat long, however, because she was on lunch at work.

As a means to calm my temper, I decided I wanted to get to work on the knitted hats I'm making for Sonia and Dean. I had seen some at the market that looked like fish, with the mouth as the rim. I thought they were hilarious and perfect for the kids, but I could not possibly spend $50 getting them.

Especially since I have the yarn to make some myself. It would mean more if I made them myself, anyway.

Sonia's favourite colours are orange and black, while Dean's is red and blue. Go figure that I have giant yarn balls of black and blue, but not red or orange. I was thinking about where I could pick up one of each colour for cheap. Then I remembered that Mum had said she had hidden a Micheal's card somewhere in my apartment (before our fight). She's done that as a means to surprise me for whenever I was doing well in school.

I went searching for the damn thing, which lead me to thinking how I could ask Mum nicely where it was at. The problem was, no matter what way I considered it, I knew I would have a fight on my hands. Which turned a mildly annoyed me when I woke up into a me that was ready to go looking for a fight.

Thankfully, I haven't text Mum. I'm hoping I will come across the card while I'm cleaning today, then I can get what I need for the kidlets' gifts.

That's not a typo, I actually refer to them as "Kidlets" and "Chijens". Words I had made up through talking too fast, and things slurring together. Which happens a lot with me. Enough that I had needed speech therapy for stuttering as a child. The words were honestly too hilarious that I decided to keep using them.

Part of me is a little worried if they would like the fish hats. Yes, they are cute and funny, but it's still a clothing article. At 7 and 4, respectively, I don't think they would enjoy them as much as a toy or chocolate. Dean is a fan of kinder eggs, though, so maybe I'll grab one for each of them to go with the hats.

It's because of those two that I'm not going to back down from my mother for Christmas. Where the adults would understand why I'd rather stay in London, the kids wouldn't. I think it would hurt Sonia way too much.

When Sonia was born, Sandra hit with a pretty hard bought of postpartum. Her difficulties did not let her be as close to Sonia as she was trying to be. That meant the baby was often handed off to someone else to care for.

At the time, I was 18, and trying to prove to myself that I could be a good motherly type. I was already a sucker around babies, but it just worked out that when Sandra handed her off, I was the one looking after Sonia. Then, when Dean came along, Sandra was clinging to him as if to compensate for lost time with Sonia. Add in the attention shift in my family that tends to happen when there's a new "youngest", and I felt horrible for poor Sonia.

I made sure I did not switch my attention like the rest. I can admit, I definitely play favourites. I try not to because it makes me worry about how I would act with my own chijens, should I ever have any. Still, I argue that Sonia needs to be someone's favourite. You can tell she's thrilled to have someone listen to her without needing to act out for attention.

It's not that I don't give Dean just as much attention. I'm just faster to react to him acting out than her. I constantly tell Sandra how I feel like a bad guy to him since I seem to be the only one telling him no, or following through with discipline (usually just taking away a toy).

I worry I'm overstepping as well. I mean, I wait for John or Sandra to say something first. I was told off once before because I had told a friend-of-the-family's children- who were rough housing- to be more gentle with each other.

I don't know, maybe it's a good thing I can't seem to have kidlets of my own. I would probably show way too much favouritism towards them, and poor Sonia would go through being cast aside again. I want to say that I would never let that happen, but I also try to tell myself that I don't play favourites when I clearly do.

Okay, this topic is making me sad. I should go do those chores I said I would do when I woke up this morning.

One of Those Moods

I'm hungry, but I have no will to eat. I'm not tired, but I want to sleep. The only reason I got through bathing today was because I needed something to calm my nerves.

Fuck, it's one of those days.

I am bored out of my mind, but anything I do, I loose interest quickly. I figured I was miserable doing fun things, being miserable while cleaning wouldn't be any different. Instead, I'm writing a bitchy little passage on my laptop.

I don't know what to do with myself. There is this bitter heat coursing just under the surface. It makes me feel sick, but that could just be that I haven't eaten yet today and barely ate yesterday.

Really, what's the point of any of it? Even when I'm trying, Mum still acts like I'm some scum of the earth, and a giant disappointment.

Fuck it all. I'll damn well message her and tell her I'm not going to Chatham for Christmas. I'd rather be miserable in the comfort of my own home than hoping nothing I say or do sets her off again.

Mr. Boomerang

I have been avoiding this topic. I know once I start, I'm going to get pissed off. Thing is, I'm already in a mood right now.

The topic in question is one Richard Burns, my biological father.

There is a part of me that wants to rip into him. A side that is still angry with him. What it comes down to is that he is nothing more than a coward. He would come around when he thought he could gain something from it, and left as soon as the pressure of being a father started.

He hurt my mother by threatening to take us from her. That was after she left his abusive ass.

He hurt me by pretending I didn't exist growing up. I'm glad for it now because I prefer to pretend he doesn't exist. It was just a sore spot as a kid.

I still remember the look on a call centre colleague of mine. I had walked into work, and she cheerily greeted me.

"Hey Annie, I saw that you and I have a mutual friend on Facebook."

"Oh yeah? Who?"

"Dawn," she said proudly. Dawn is my step-mother, and mother to my three youngest siblings.

"Oh, cool," I cheerfully responded, not thinking anything of it. I like Dawn. I can't fault her for getting mixed up with Richard. The guy can sure put on a show as some noble, and considerate human being. Complete bullshit, but that's a con artist for you.

That's also why she was among my friends list, and he was blocked. It wouldn't stop him from seeing my posts, because he could just use her, or one of the kids', accounts. Still, I knew it was probably grinding his gears.

"How do you know her and Dick?" Robin's question had been so innocent. I knew she had to be one of those people that he was pulling the wool over.

I actually stopped on my way to my desk, which was down the row from her, to look at her, face to face, "Richard's my father."

She looked like I was trying to tell her the moon was made of cheese.

One of my friends, I can't remember if it was Lynn or Kendra that said it, had to break the sudden tension I felt with, "Oh boy. That just opened up a can of worms!"

The team and I laughed. Robin, despite being down the row from me, still had to comment. "I didn't know he had other children."

I had heard that line about a dozen times before.

"Yeah, he likes to act like my sister and I don't exist unless he can warp it to make himself look good."

Which is true. I have even called him out on it.

For example. Growing up, I was rather close with his sister, my Aunt Carly. She was the one that allowed me to grow in faith, because, despite being baptized Catholic, no one on my mother's side of the family practices. To be honest, there's been more than a few occasions Mum has referred to religious people as yahoos, forgetting she was insulting me while doing so.

Still, I had met God through church in my Catholic school. I wanted to continue a relationship with Him, and there was a double bonus that it gave me a chance to be around my aunt, Uncle Jim, and my cousins (and eventually my cousin's children).

Aunt Carly used to run the Sunday School activities. I was too old for her groups age range, but she let me stay as one of her helpers. That meant I knew the church, and a lot of it's people already. I had to stop going for a while after I came home one Sunday school, and decided my favourite TV show was opening me to the influences of the devil.

I REALLY held a high value in the things my aunt said at that point in time.

Mum freaked out. I realized when I got older that she was just scared I wasn't thinking for myself. Which, at that point in time, I wasn't. That may be why she still seems to think I'm incredibly impressionable. Maybe I am, to some degree. I'd like to think that I'm not.

Richard was also a regular at that particular church. I stayed far away from him when I could, but being a Sunday School helper let me spend time with my siblings. While I was at the church, Aunt Carly made sure everyone was aware that I was her niece, and Richard my father. It forced Richard to play up the kind and loving father that had done wrong, and was just looking for forgiveness.

By that point, it had to be about his third or fourth time giving me that spiel. I was weary, but my forgiving nature was still foolishly willing to give him a chance.

With a wide birth between us when I could help it, anyway.

When I no longer went to that church thanks to my episode, he didn't talk to me. In fact, when I was old enough to say I wanted to go back, there were a lot of new people. None of them knew Richard had been with someone outside of Dawn. What a surprise to learn he had two other children, all over again. Of course, he had to play up his charade, again. Except there were enough people from before to notice, and didn't question me on why I was so cold towards him.

The last time I had seen him was before my 19th birthday. Life was starting to get busy, so I didn't have the time to go to church as often as I wanted to. Not to mention, Mum was getting fairly vicious with some of her comments. That's why I started to practice in private.

I have to give Richard credit for trying to keep up with me. I think he had learned his lesson from just letting things drop last time. I woke up the Saturday of my 19th birthday with a message from him. The gist of it was,

"Happy 19th Birthday. I'm so proud of the woman you've grown up to be."

It pissed me off. Mum had kept the same phone number so that he was free to call us during our birthdays, and holidays. She kept the line open, and didn't even say anything bad about him until we were old enough to figure him out for ourselves. He never did. Not even during the years that he was talking to us.

I knew what the game was. Father's Day was the 20th, that year. He was probably hoping I'd be so grateful for the well wishes that I would provide my own. Which would show he was just the greatest father ever.

I was not having it. I came back with a private message, "Well, 1 out of 14 isn't bad, but I guess it's better late than never. I should say thank you, anyway, because my MOTHER raised me to be polite. So, thanks, and take care."

Mum wouldn't stop grinning when I told her.

The priceless bit was his come-back. "Wow, 19 years old, and still such a child. Well, I guess I'll wish you all your Happy Birthdays, and Merry Christmases. Oh, and congratulations on your wedding, too. Since I'm sure I won't be invited to that! Have a good life without me to drag you down."

That was overnight, so I didn't get it until the next morning. Mum and I were laughing up a storm. Seriously, I am childish, but I can admit it. He, on the other hand... Does he even know the phrase, "the pot calling the kettle black"?

I mean, the part about my wedding didn't make sense to me, since I wasn't engaged. Now that I think about it, I think it's because I was dating Nick at the time, and he must have known. Still, if I ever do get married, there is no fucking way he's walking me down the isle. My mother is doing that!

I went to check if he had posted some pathetic update on his page in hopes of people sympathizing with him. That was when I discovered he had blocked me. I just laughed harder. I swear, I had tears in my eyes.

By the way, Mum and I went for ice cream afterwards to celebrate (my request).

About a year later, I noticed I could see his comment on one of the kids' posts. I figured he was trying to keep tabs to swindle a way out of having to pay child support. He had been doing as much since I was little. Mum still has the letter outlining how he had applied in the courts to have Nicholas officially adopt us, so long as he was left off the hook about paying. That was less than a year into Mum and Nicholas' relationship.

That was when I blocked him. Not because there was anything that he could use, but because I figured it would annoy him to no end. I wish I could say that was the last I heard from him, but it wasn't.

A couple years ago, he decided to up and leave his wife and children. The youngest was 12 years old, at the time. He moved out to BC, which pissed me off. Here I had been saving up to go there for film school, and now I had to wonder if I would accidentally run into him. I figured it was a big enough city, though, so I kept trying anyway. I know he had spent time there because he was supposed to take care of one of his brothers. I don't know that uncle, and I'm doubtful Richard actually did anything to help. He wasn't the type to lift a finger for Dawn and the kids, either.

He must have met some woman while he was there, because he was dating shortly after leaving Ontario. Tiffany, the only of the children that was not his by blood, had moved out there with him for school. With her out there, he could not pretend he didn't have previous offspring. I heard this other chick has two boys of her own, as well. I assume to impress her, and make her believe that his poor relationship was because of us instead of him, he sent the other four of us a message in March of last year.

It was a "poor pity me" message where he pointed blame at his parents being too old when they had had him, and they died when he was still so young. I wish I still had the message somewhere around here so I could quote it. It was utter rubbish, where he was saying sorry, but not meaning a word of it. To bring his dead parents into it was a new low for him, to boot.

I don't know for sure if my brother, Noah, or Dawn had said anything back in response. Cam, our youngest sister, Maria, me, and Mum (who had been informed by Cam) sure as Hell did. I had been at work when Cam texted me that he had had Tiffany send us all a message. It gave me time to simmer down before responding. Unlike Cam, Maria, and Mum, who were all at him in a heart beat with verbal claws at the ready.

Granted, my co-workers sure got an earful.

He actually had the nerve to come back at Mum, saying it was none of her business. Except, it very much is her business when it involves HER daughters. Her message had been a simple, "You fucked up, and they don't want you in their lives" sort of thing.

My response though, thanks to having the chance to calm and think clearly, was that of cold fire. Richard is the only person that has gained such a level of loathing from me. I've come to shake off stupidity that is directed at me. I cope, and try to move on. No one, however, hurts my siblings, or speaks so disrespectfully to my mother. Even now, as I remember this, I can feel the heat rising just under my skin.

As calmly as I could muster, I clearly outlined to him that he was no father of mine. I told him that I did pity him, but not for the dumb reasons he had wrote. I pitied him because he was a coward that would forever be on the run. Wherever he goes, people will come to see him for who he is, and hate and shun him for it. When he is old, and alone, he will have no one to blame for it but himself.

He's going to leave behind a trail of people who despise him. Thankfully, Dawn mentioned she had convinced him to be snipped, so there won't be more Burns children out there being hurt by his selfish ways.

Needless to say, I didn't get a response to that. I hope he's finally gotten the picture, and will stay out of my life.

He's the one person that I don't think I can ever forgive. I tried when I was little, and it backfired at me. Lately, I've tried, again, for the sake of my own piece of mind, and a lot of my anger has turned to pity. I'm learning that you can forgive someone, and not allow yourself to be open to them to be hurt again.

He has no place in my future. Not even the memory of him. Thus, he will be staying here, and out of my thoughts. I know there is so much more I can say about him, but I am washing my hands of the matter.

After all, Mum taught me to always be the bigger person, and walk away.

Hope

I love my Aunt Heather. Truly. If there is anyone that can calm me down, and actually talk to me like an adult, it's her. I sent her a message earlier saying that I don't want to come home for Christmas. She called me just a few minutes ago to talk me through it.

She knows the way my mother can be, and understands why I didn't want to go. She also didn't want me to be sad and alone on Christmas day. She did ask me if the reason I didn't want to go was because I was spending Christmas with Nick. Which I'm not.

It was fun being able to talk to her about Nick, and know that it's not going back to my mother. She agrees that it's none of Mum's business who I talk to, or see, or whatever. She admitted that she had to be the one to help Mum find out what the number was since I never actually put Nick's name in my contacts (back when Mum snooped through my phone in August).

Here's the kicker, though. Turns out, the reason Heather was able to figure out who the number belong to was because he had put up a sex ad. I just searched to see if it was still up. It's not, but I'll be keeping an eye out just in case.

Oh, and I passed all my classes. I only got a 50% on all of them, and I'm on academic probation, but I've survived. Now I have to wait with my meeting with Anita on the 4th to figure out next semester.

At last, I can breathe.

New semester. New start. It's not going to be easy, but I'm hopeful.

You know what, I think I'm actually going to work on my novel for a little bit.

Home For the Holidays

It's Christmas afternoon. In my family, the holiday party doesn't start until dinner. I have a few moments of quiet to actually sit and write.

I did come back to Chatham for Christmas. It was even my mother that picked me up, and who I am staying with. She had called me on the 22nd, asking me "how badly did I want to come home that night".

I didn't want to at all. I was hoping she would have held off until her day off on the 24th, or, at least, until she was done work on the 23rd. Either would have been less time here. I tried to play up that it was up to her, and what would be more convenient. She kept saying that someone told her there would be a storm on the 23rd, so it would be safer to go tonight.

I'm pretty sure it was an excuse. I know that she would prefer to drive in the day, instead of when it's dark. By the time she had left Chatham, it was already 5:30 pm by the time she reached London. That late, and the fact she had to work in the morning, there was no point for her to come get me then. Except for someone to be there to watch her dogs.

Mum even called me on her lunch break to make sure I was awake to let her dogs outside. That way she didn't have to run home on her break. She can spend that time playing Pokemon Go, instead.

I will give Mum some credit. It took twenty minutes before she started in on "why she was angry" and wording things in a way that made it sound like I should feel guilty. She even made a point that, according to her, the reason she had a sore neck and shoulder was because she was so stressed that Saturday.

"It's probably because I was clenching the wheel. The only solace I had was knowing that Grandpa was driving behind me. Until I had to stop for gas in Thamesville. Then they waved at me as they passed. So I called Heather. Just so I had someone on the phone while I was getting through all that shit."

Yeah, except Cam told me the weather had not been that bad the very same night. According to her, the roads were not even slick.

Also, Mum had called Heather earlier than that. She would have called regardless of the weather just to play the poor her, and what an ungrateful little bitch I am. I know this, because she has done so repeatedly. A lot of times, I was still in hearing distance while she complained about, and belittled, me.

Ask me why I have self-esteem issues...

Regardless, I don't feel guilty. I was getting annoyed, instead. I fired right back at her, in her same tone, about how I had to or else I would have failed one of my classes. I would have failed all of them, honestly, but I wasn't telling her that.

It got the point across that I was not going to budge about the issue. Eventually, she stopped bringing it up.

As for her sore neck and shoulder, we made a stop to play Pokemon as soon as we got in town. She went to look at her phone, hissed with pain, and then looked at me with a smirk.

"I wonder if that's what's causing me issues. I'm playing too much Pokemon that I'm cricking my neck wrong." She then laughs, "How many people can say they have a Pokemon Go injury?"

So much for the muscle stress being my fault. Honestly...

I did manage to keep my cool as well, though. See, earlier that day on the 22nd, I had had a meeting with Linda. I told her about Mum's attitude the 17th, and the eggshells I had been walking on for those couple days before.

She looked me dead in the eye, "It sounds like she's a very unpredictable woman. That must be a high stress environment to be in."

I couldn't have agreed more with that statement.

"You know that is emotional abuse, right?"

I nodded. I know better than to say that in front of my mother, though. Cam did once, and Mum just added it to her arsenal to prove how she has such horrible, and ungrateful children.

I openly admitted to Linda, "When Mum get's stressed, her personality turns toxic. She's quick to shoot you down when you're happy about something, and any little thing will set her off."

"And that's not your fault," Linda insisted. "You can't control the way your mother is, or make excuses for her. All you can do is control how you react to it."

We disused some counter measures, which I had plenty of. I'm not new to this dance. Then Linda pressed me for preventative measures. She convinced me to spend Friday with my sister instead of hiding in the room where I was at Mum's mercy. That's why, as soon as I left the meeting, I text Cam. The trade off was, I did have to let her dye my hair.

Cam and I have been getting on well for the last month. The paranoid part of me wants to ruin it by thinking she's just doing it for Christmas so that I'll get her something nice.

What she did for me, however, negates that feeling.

She was far too excited to wait the two days until Christmas to give me my gift. After a couple minutes of pleading, I caved.

The majority of the things she gave me were hand made, *Harry Potter* themed items like a Hogwarts letter, and a hand made wand. There was even mason jars with "potions" labelled on them. Turns out there were shampoo, soap, and bubble bath.

You'd think the kid knows how much I love home-spa treating myself, or something. I was speechless.

My favourite of these cleverly made gifts however was

the box of candy. It looks to be a shoe box that's been covered with Santa wrapping paper, and stuffed full of sweets. The best part about that, however, was that she had stuck a little piece of paper on the lid that read, "In case of Dementor attack, open IMMEDATELY."

I couldn't stop laughing the moment I saw it. I'm keeping that damn box next to my desk at home. That's where I'm going to keep any and all of my candy from now on, and my girls had better not tear off the label.

There were two store bought items. The first was a windows tablet. I own an apple one that Mum had given me a couple years back, but it had been knocked (not by me, surprisingly) from my bed onto hardwood floor. The screen has a giant spider's web crack throughout it. Not enough to make it unusable, but still enough for people to cringe upon seeing the poor beat up thing.

Which is why the one my sister gave me includes a protective cover.

It was honestly the most generous of gifts she could have given me. I found out after that it cost over $100. That's a small fortune to both Cam and I. I was happy with the homemade stuff, and the sturdy backpack it all came in. She said that everyone seemed to be having a shitty year, and so she wanted to treat us.

I know it's not a competition, but it really made me feel like crap that I couldn't do more for her back. The materials I used to make her wall hanging Kitsune mask had been squirrelled away from leftovers in my sculpture class. The end result was no bigger than my hand.

Oops, it's 4:30, and Mum is waking up. I'll be sure to write more, after I get home from family Christmas.

Morning Musings

I have no idea how I'm awake at 7:30 am on boxing day. For one thing, I have officially learned that my drink of choice involves pop and amaretto liquor. As long as that pop isn't fruit flavoured. I had attempted to see what *Grape Crush* mixed with half a shot of amaretto would taste like.

Cough syrup. It tasted like fucking cough syrup.

I had finish a little over half of the mickey by the end of the night. That's far more than I have ever done in a single evening. Thankfully, the end of the night was midnight, so I was able to sip, and not get more than a little heated in the cheeks at any given point.

Which is the other point. After the party was done, grandma still wanted to play some Pokemon Go. Thus, I did not return to my mother's house until after 2:30 am.

That is why I am saying, I have no idea how I'm this alert, this early in the morning. I've actually been fighting to go back to sleep since 6. The lovely combination of acid reflux and dehydration had been the reason I woke up to begin with. I wouldn't claim to be hungover, but I definitely have a minor headache, and don't trust burps or hiccups, at the moment.

I suppose I was doing what I could to relax, but also stay alert the entire time. My sister was in a "bitch at any little thing" kind of mood. For whatever reason, that meant I was on her shit list. Nearly two hours into the night, and I was pissed off with her, and couldn't enjoy my limited time with OUR family because I had to watch for her random attacks.

Mum wasn't much better. We were having fun, just like last Saturday with Grandma's side of the family. Then, as 9:30 pm rolled around, I was not ready to leave yet. Mum was insisting I was to go with her. She was apparently sore again. The plan was that she wanted me to put this electric muscle shocker thing on her back for her. I don't know what it is, just that it uses little shocks to force muscles to relax.

She was not asking for me to put the device on her, either. She never just asks for help with anything. It's one of my pet peeves. I'm a very helpful person, and need little prompting to jump to another's aid. I just ask that you be respectful enough to ask, instead of telling me that I'm doing something with the expectation I'll do it.

I suppose it's my own fault. I've never actually told Mum "no" when she 'asks' me to do something for her. Just the other night, she said, "I think I'm going to have you put vitarub on my shoulder for me."

I did it for her because she needed it, but I was as annoyed as a hornets nest that some kid decided was a pinata.

That's what Mum was doing again last night. It was the usual reasons why she needed to leave, followed up with, "When we get home, you can put (whatever the device is called) on me."

I, for one, certainly didn't feel like dropping everything like some servant because master wants something.

Thankfully, Cam dropped the attitude long enough to help in my defence towards staying. "Grandma and I can drop her off. I'm sure we'll be out later."

I even offered up a compromise. I figured her littlest dog would bark his head off, and wake her when I got in, so I could put it on her then.

"No, I just won't do it tonight," was her snarky answer.

She put up very little fight to me staying after that. She did however make sure to play up how 'hurt' she was as she got ready... and then carried the bin with her gifts in it into the van just fine; despite people offering to help. Boy, you've really convinced me that you're injured, and I'm being selfish and ungrateful, again.

Wow, not sure if I'm in a mood this morning, or if this is just legitimate annoyance with what I'm writing. I'm going to try to get more sleep while I can. Mum will be home from work by 2:30 pm, and will likely be on my ass if I'm still sleeping then.

I mean, her conure still yells my name when she comes home because that's what she used to do when I lived there.

I just hope Grandma does decide to visit after she drops Cam at work for 11 AM. We'll see.

After Christmas Calm-down

A quarter to midnight. It's arranged that I'll be dropped off back to London by my grandparents instead of waiting on my mother to decided when she feels like it. I wouldn't put it past her to make me wait an extra day, just because. She's probably still harbouring a grudge from Yolanda's party.

I got to hang out with John, Sandra, and the kids again today. Us adults were searching for music videos on youtube on the TV since my bored scrolling through available ringtones got us on the topic of songs. I came to learn that Mum is a fan of Pentatonix, like I am. Plus, the reason Sonia had started learning violin was because she had been watching my favourite violinist, Lindsey Sterling, online.

Speaking of the kidlets, they ended up loving their hats. At one point Sonia stretched the toque-fish over her face, and started to chase her brother. Dean eventually did the same, and the pair played this game of "fish monster chase" against one another. Don't worry, they could clearly see and breathe through the knitted holes.

So, at last, the holiday stress is over.

Normally, it would last until the 27th, because that was when we would have to deal with Grandpa's side of the family. That, at long last, has been cancelled though.

I have nothing against my extended family. It's just, the last couple of times we tried to get together for Christmas, my grandfather's three children and their families try to make all the plans without including us. Only to complain when we try to make the plans instead. Add in the fact we don't seem to exist to them for the rest of the year, nor wish their own father a happy birthday, or happy father's day.... There is just too much miss-communication, and questions of if we are considered family.

I mean, there was one time my Aunt introduced me to her

son's new girlfriend as, "My step-sister's daughter." That had pissed off Mum far more than it did me. Don't call me her niece, or anything to personal like that.

I might write a passage about all this another time, but, for now, it's time to get some sleep.

Sonia had picked out a gift for me too. It's a wooden sign to hang on my wall that reads: Wizards Welcome (Muggles Tolerated). That's getting hung on my Wall of Personality as soon as I get home.

I don't know if I've mentioned my wall before. It's beside my desk with various things meant to make me smile on it. There's:

A stylized portrait of "The Statue of David"'s head.

Some inspirational plaques.

A picture of Mum and I, laughing together, that my sister had taken. It's one of few professional pictures which Mum is genuinely smiling in it.

An 11x17 poster of one of my novel's potential covers (since I had paid to have it made a year ago).

And, lastly, a sign Nelly had given me that says, "Warning: Novelist at work. Bystanders may be written into the story."

Now I have Sonia's sign to add to the collection.

Nothing to Prove

It's 2 am on the 30th. I haven't had a lot to write about that required reflecting over these last couple of days. Which, once I realized that, caused me to reflect on the matter.

Because there's nothing dangerous about over-thinking things, what so ever.

Thankfully, my mind is currently at peace. I had a good time with my family, save for minor annoyances. I'm comfortable at home with food in my belly, and warm clothes to wear. I've even been consistently cleaned, which really helps the self-esteem.

When I came home on the 27th, I actually wanted to clean. My floors have been swept, and my Christmas items neatly packed away for next year's use. I've folded a fair amount of my clothes too, instead of letting them rest in a basket.

For the first time in a while, I just feel peaceful. I know the majority of it is simply how the Christmas season effects me in positive ways. Still, I hope I can make it last.

There are a couple small things, though, that are helping as well. The first being my new mantra, since my meeting on the 22nd with Linda:

I have nothing to prove to anyone but myself.

It helped me get through some of my annoyances with my family. Not only did I not have anything to prove to them, but they didn't have anything to prove to me. I'm not my mother, or sister, or grandmother, and they are not me. There shouldn't be standards, or expectations. We're all just going to be us.

Which then lead me to remember something one of my grade 7 teachers had said.

I only had him for one class a week (Social studies, I think). We had been told to do a project in which we were given a country to make a pamphlet brochure on. It would require a lot of research, but the final result was simple.

I was at an age where I was content handing in this half-done, shotty piece of paper. I couldn't be bothered to put any pride in my schoolwork. Not like when I was younger.

I almost wonder if that was a sign of my health declining, or simply teenaged angst.

Either way, I'm pretty sure there had been some procrastinating involved, as well. He set us to work on something else while he called us up, one by one. He had taken one look at mine, and said, "Are you proud of handing this into me?"

"I tried my best," I shrugged.

"I don't want you to *try* your best. I asked you to *do* your best," he coolly countered.

I didn't understand the difference then. Couple days ago, that saying just popped into my head. I mulled it over, and realized that what Linda was telling me was the same thing as my teacher had been saying.

I am me. As long as I do my best, no one can fault me for it. No one can ask more; not even me. Even if it takes me a long time to get where I want to be. There may be those that feel they need to sneer, and criticize, but I don't answer to them. They don't answer to me, either. At the end of the day, I must live with my choices, and only God has the right to judge me.

In less than 48 hours, a new year is coming. I have another chance at school, in a program I enjoy. Where will I go after? I have no idea. I want to write, though. I always want to write. I want to entertain, and delight. I want to make people happy, but it's likely I won't do that for every soul I touch. And that's perfectly fine. I will just keep doing my best.

I know I'm hopeful now. It's going to be a question of how I react when life takes a swing at me.

Still, I'm not going to let my inner turmoil take that from me. I will breathe, be patient, and take each day as it comes.

Melancholy

It is officially 2017.

Not really sure how I feel right now. On the one hand, I'm glad for the end of one rough year, and starting fresh on one with a little more hope. I have no idea how good or bad this is going to go, but I'm not letting myself worry.

I was exceptionally lonely today. It could be the combination of boredom and isolation. I've been using my wii games, and new andriod box to distract myself, but I don't feel mentally excited. It's made me consider actually going to my mother's on the 4th. Except, I have no intention of staying with her another 4 days, either.

Still, I did reach out to Mum, Heather, and Cam when the loneliness was growing overwhelming. Turns out, Mum was working, so she didn't answer back until after 10:30. Heather didn't answer at all, but that was not as bad as my sister answering.

I straight up told her I was lonely at the beginning of our texts. She proceeds to rub in how great it is that she's at a party with HER friends. Oh, but wait, she's uncomfortable now because there are two strangers that are friends with HER friends. I got annoyed with her complaining about these other people's presence. I told her that she should enjoy the fact she's around friends, and then excused myself.

Later, she text me to let me know about a friend of hers from Barrie. She told me to send him a message and see about hanging out since he was "super nerdy, and loves DnD". Oh, and he lives in London now. I figured it was someone to talk to about games.

He did tell me about a place called the Cardboard Cafe. I looked it up. It's not far from me, and it's literally a cafe with hundreds of board games to play. I had considered going tonight, but then got stuck in a movie.

The movie finished up shortly before midnight, so I curled up in bed. Cleo came in to cuddle with me just as the shouting and fireworks started. I didn't get up to watch them. I merely to attempted to sleep. Of course, I woke up at 2 am.

I got up, and lite a candle. It was a gift from my mother during Christmas. I've been using it as my only light source for the last three nights; save for whatever electronic device I'm messing with. The tiny, flickering glow usually sends me into one of my 'poetic' moods. Not really sure how else to describe it.

It's a sort of artistic mindset, as any little thing sparks inspiration and fresh ideas. At the same time, I'm lulled and mellow. Not quiet in a state of peace, but certainly one of calm. I get this way around campfires, too. I have no idea why.

I considered hopping onto my computer now to write more of my novel. Except, even under the candle light, I'm indifferent. I know writing will improve my mood, which is why I started by writing this passage. Yet, I can't be bothered.

Just as I can't be bothered to cook a half-decent meal to fill my grumbling stomach.

Or how I want, dearly, to have a hot bubble bath, but don't care enough to run the water.

I have games to play, and movies to watch. So, why haven't I turned a single one on?

I think the word that describes me today is "melancholy". Allow me a moment to check my dictionary to be sure.

Well, that's ironic. I always understood melancholy to mean apathetic, and/or indifferent. Maybe with a hint of sadness thrown in. I had not expected the definition to straight out be, "a gloomy state of mind, especially when habitual or prolonged; depression".

Fucking great. I'm starting my new year in the throngs of a depression spell. I should have baked cupcakes earlier, like I had considered. I generally feel good while baking or cooking.

I just detest the clean up, afterwards.

I just have no desire to make more dishes when I'm already struggling to get done the ones I already have. I've made some progress in cleaning them, but there is still a pan or two that I'm sure has been there since before Christmas.

I hate it. I hate looking at it, and the smell of it. It makes me think of Mum's words about how lazy I am. If she came to visit, it'd be the first thing she would be on my ass about. I know it's going to get fruit flies, and mold if I leave it any longer. I also know to actually clean it is going to be atrocious when I finally get the will to tackle it.

You know, I just remembered the time Mum had wanted to cancel Christmas because the dishes were not done. It was while both Cam and I lived with her. The two of use would be given a set amount of chores to have done before Mum got home from work.

She never said who was to do what chore. She would name off the list before heading out to work, or over a phone call. I wish she would have wrote it down so nothing would be forgotten. Or she could yell at us saying something was forgotten when it had never been mentioned.

Heck, you'd think one too many time being yelled at for forgetfulness I would have learned to write shit down myself.

The point is, Cam and I were to decide for ourselves who did what. Most of the time, I did the majority, and then had to argue with Cam to get hers done. She had this attitude that Mum was going to yell at both of us, anyway.

Which Mum did. Even if I named off all the things I had single-handedly done, it wasn't good enough. Her attention was on what wasn't done. Plus, as the oldest, I should be more responsible than that.

The worst was the dishes. Too often, it would get put off until just before Mum got home. Which, naturally, was the trigger to one of her fits.

It was a chore that one of us would wash and the other dry one time, and the opposite next. Eventually, Cam started to "leave a pan to soak" if she didn't want to wash it. If she was being particularly lazy, the pan would be put into the sink with still more sitting on the counter. I would turn around, and leave the same pan/dishes so that she had to clean them. Which would piss Mum off.

The result was that, if one of us should leave a dish, we would have to wash the next load. That lead to arguments about who's turn it actually was. I didn't want to roll over to my sister, but I also wanted to make sure Mum didn't have a reason to yell at us when she got home.

That didn't matter if Mum was working a double shift, however. On those days, our assigned chores were not enough. Only an absolutely spotless house would appease her. Something the pair of us had no desire to even attempt.

Needless to say, it was very stressful life under any given day.

So, lets add a double shift on Christmas Eve. My sister and I arguing about who's turn it was to get the dishes done. Which resulted in them not being washed by the time Mum came in the door.

Mum is screaming, "Why does it take me getting pissed off for either of you to get off your lazy asses, and help me? I just worked fifteen fucking hours. I actually thought about how nice it'll be to come home to wrap gifts for you guys, and now I have to do the fucking dishes."

Of course, Cam and I had been through the routine enough to know we were not to say a word. Any back talk would make it worse. Just as glaring resulted in being grounded for a week; no matter which of us that did the glare.

There is also the point that if a chore was not completed before Mum got home, or not done to her standard, she would do it in front of us, complaining the entire time. I once tried to cut in to vacuum the couch better; since I apparently hadn't done it good enough the first time. She shoved me away. Not a full push, but more of a side check to get me out of the way.

"I said I'll fucking do it myself!"

Also, heaven forbid Cam and I walked away from one of her rants. She would just scream louder, for longer, and threaten to take our bedroom doors. I remember my sister's door being off it's hinges for a few days.

Funny enough, Mum wouldn't do it herself when it came to the dishes. She would scream her fit, and then we were to do them then and there.

That night was not the case. As she screamed about us being useless, she hit a new breaking point.

"Fine! We just won't have fucking dishes since you guys are ruining them all anyway!" Then she grabbed the sink full of plates and such, and threw them in the trash. Cam and I were forced to pick them out, and clean them, later on. I remember having to be super careful because one plate shattered into pieces. There are some of Mum's mugs that had chips and cracks in them. I don't know if she got rid of them, however.

After throwing out the dishes, she started in on part two of her rants: how ungrateful we were to her. "You know what? We're not fucking having Christmas. I'm just going to return everything to the stores. It'll sure save me a shit ton of money."

She ended up getting over her attitude by the time she had finished her 6:30 to 2:30 shift the following day. The dishes were cleaned, and we had been put in our places, again. Time for the 'apology' part of the cycle.

Yet, as I have said before, no one in my family apologizes. In Mum's case, she just gives us stuff, or acts like nothing was wrong and just laughs and jokes. Of course, there are a lot of times she doesn't get to this stage for a week, at least. In the mean time, we're on eggshells because anything, great or small, could set her off again, and prolong the stress.

She came home, hid upstairs, and wrapped everything. Then had us bring it all downstairs to be opened. I'm sure there are pictures of us not quiet as jolly as we usually are for Christmas. Still, we made the best of it.

You know, it actually feels good to get this out there. I can remember so many times I would tell myself, "I was not abused. I'm just lazy, or don't know how to do things right". Thing is, looking back, there were a lot of times my mother was abusive to me. The saddest part is, she doesn't even do it on purpose. She has no more control over it than I do this depression spell I'm in.

I think I just needed to vent out some frustrations for a little bit. Let's hope this won't need to be a trend in this new year.

Also, Happy New Year to me. I discovered I still had one can of Ginger Ale hidden in the back of my fridge. Looks like I still get to treat myself for my first full night of the new year. I'm going to enjoy my pop, and go watch something on Netflix. Maybe a kid's movie since they are light-hearted and fun.

Day One in Pantanal

Nick has just left my place to head to work. I wasn't expecting him to visit last night, but he had text me from outside my door. I couldn't think of a nice way to tell him I wasn't in the mood for what his sexual text messages indicated. I was glad for the company, though.

It's one of the reasons that I will be going back to Chatham tomorrow. I need to get out and socialize, even if it means being under my mother's thumb for four days. We are going to buy a few groceries, though, so there is that bonus.

None of that is why I wanted to write this morning. I was considering starting in on my novel. Problem was, I was quiet comfortable in my bed with a warm body pressed against my back. Odd, because normally the extra heat makes me uncomfortable. Instead, it did lull me into a calm state of mind.

It was while I listened to his gentle snoring, and starred at the blank grey sky outside, I started to think about Brazil.

Sometimes, like now, I fondly think about it, and grow homesick. I know what I'm really feeling is a longing for adventure.

Wander lust, someone once told me.

Brazil was a turning point in my life. People kept telling me that it was an opportunity of a lifetime. That statement had not truly sunk in until I was a little older. It was a time that I just felt alive over the course of a hundred moments. I felt free, and nearly every day was something new. The moment that began this train of thought was my first morning in Pantanal.

First, let me clear up one common mistake revolving around Brazil. Their first language is Portuguese, not Spanish. Keep that in mind, because "Pantanal" is a Portuguese word. One that I snicker at each time I say it in relation to the place I visited. For now, let's just say someone was being a very literal smart-ass when they named it.

It was first of the three trips available to exchange students to explore the country in greater depth. The second trip was far too expensive, and I came home before the third was available.

There were only two states that were south from Pantanal, and Paraná, the state I resided in, was one of them. Thus we exchange student had been divided between two tour groups. The 8 of us from the South, and the other 30 or so from the North. It was a long drive, and our two groups congregated together at a hotel just outside of Pantanal. My group got there first, allowing us time to settle in, and play in the pool before the horde came in.

The first hotel had been awesome, and fun, resulting in yours truly conking out early. It meant that for the entire trip, I was one of the first to sleep, and first to rise.

The following morning, the lot of us were rounded up onto a large bus. Then drove several hours to get to our destination. By the time we got there, it was dark, and dinner time.

I could tell coming off the bus that we were super close to nature. There was a lack of man-made noise pollution, and the air was crisp, and clean. My senses came alive, and I was curious about what was out there. I could not see what was beyond the fence, however, as the lamps were only enough to see the walk way to get from the sleeping quarters to the dinning hall.

There was no time to explore either. Which I later learned was a good thing. We were ushered off to supper, held in an open air room. There were no glass windows, anywhere, by the way. There were screens to keep out the bugs, but closing up meant large wooden shutters.

As for the bedroom, in a word, it was cozy. There were two single beds, and one bunk bed, with barely enough room for a person to walk between them. Yes, we did sleep four girls in that room. I took the top bunk, being the adult-child that I am. After dinner, but before bed, there had to be six of us in there, laughing and carrying on.

I have a picture of the tiny girl from Finland, where her face is beat red. She's grinning ear to ear, and her head hanging off the side of the bed. If any of my pictures describe how crazy we were being, it's that one. I see it, and I remember being in the exact same state.

With happily filled bellies, a long trip, and finally getting the chance to expel excess energy, we were all exhausted. I wasn't the first to bed that night, but I had to be a close fifth.

Then came the morning. My ears perked to the buzz of bird song outside. The first wisps of grey light was peaking through the shutter cracks. I didn't want to disturb my roommates, but I couldn't get myself to go back to sleep. I was much too excited to get out there, and see what there was.

I slipped down the ladder, hoping that I was not shaking the bunk enough to bother the Taiwanese girl sleeping on the bottom. I can't remember if I had woke her or not. I hurriedly got ready, grabbed my camera, and was out the door in minutes. Boy, was I glad that I did.

"Pantanal" means "Swamp" or "Marshland". Beyond the fence was exactly that; a gorgeous marsh with a pool of water mere feet away.

We were actually surrounded by swamp on all sides, save for the bridge road, and the area within the fence where the hotel was resting.

The sky was alight was the rising sun, casting the tropical trees in a heavenly glow. The more the sun climbed higher into the sky, the more songs filled the air. I snapped several pictures that I still prize to this day. In my opinion, it was the most beautiful sunrise I had ever witnessed.

I had wanted to go to the other side of the fence to get a

picture of the reflection off the water. Thing is, this was swamp land in Brazil. I had wanted to be a zoologist for the longest time before I started writing. I knew well enough what could be lurking just under the surface. As pretty as it was, I respectfully kept my distance.

An hour later, the ground keeper comes out with a large, plastic basin. By then, some of the others had pulled themselves from bed. They had missed out on the sunrise, but it was still early enough for the evening cool to kiss any exposed skin. I kid you not, as the grounds keeper slips through the wire of the fence, a girl that I had gained somewhat of a friendship with (from America) asked where all the alligators were.

Then the keeper starts hitting the side of the basin with a stick like a breakfast bell. The once calm pool comes to life with half a dozen gators looking to be fed. I didn't know that what he was feeding them was piranha. Not until we went fishing on the last day, and caught the gators food for them.

I found out that he was feeding them so that they would be less likely to take one of his horses, or oxes. I didn't know he was keeping either on the grounds until later when we went horse back riding through the marsh. Turns out, the hotel doubled as a farm, and the ox mostly ran free.

To be honest, Brazil was the last time I can say I felt confident in myself. It took courage to face down the rotary people during the screening process. Then more bravery to get on a plane for the first time. Especially without any of my family with me. Then travel somewhere to spend months immersed in a culture I knew almost nothing about.

But then I came home early. I started shaping my life according to Nick's dreams. Over time, I lost sight of who I was. All that remains are the pictures and memories. Small moments. Perhaps this homesickness is also a desire for a touch of that courage and confidence I once had. Maybe, in the future, I should plan a short visit, and see if it helps. For now, it's back to bed so I have energy for today's errands.

In Case of Emergency

I certainly can't say that my life is boring. To back up some, there was this morning. I couldn't seem to fall asleep until after 9 am, when I had wanted to be up and moving by 10. This resulted in me fighting with my alarm until I absolutely had to get up for my appointment at the school. The appointment was for 2 pm.

Anita pulled it off again. Not only did she use a single hour to assign what classes I'll be attending this winter, but apparently the first of these classes starts tomorrow. Which meant that I had to cancel on Mum about returning to Chatham.

The downside of my registration is that I had to go to the registration office to have everything set. Except, this is when the international students arrived to do their winter term registration. Yep, that was a very long wait; approximately 2 hours, in fact.

I didn't get done even half of my errands for today. I was exhausted by the time I dragged myself home, but had to pay bills. Only to realize I had exactly enough for rent and bills, but nothing for groceries. Thus, I had to debate whether I go to a food bank, or, break the first rule I had made when I intentionally signed up for school: ask to borrow from Mum.

Turns out, e-transferring $30 is pretty straight forward. Who knew.

Mum says I don't have to worry about paying her back, but it still bothers me. It also means that she now has an idea of exactly how financially strapped I am. I've been rather aloof when she asks. I know it's going to cause her to worry, so hopefully Anita can work some more magic, and get me into the program we briefly talked about during today's meeting. One that's supposed to help me get an on campus job. Yes, the job will carry over the summer, too.

It would be nice to be making a living, again. I've felt, and have been treated, like a leach on the system for too long.

Anyway, the point of all this is to understand why I was dead-asleep at 9 pm... when the building's fire alarm started to go off.

I will give my anxiety one piece of credit. When I initially moved out of my mother's house, I constantly worried about how do I save my cats in case of a fire. It caused me to hold onto Mum's cat carrier for a long time. Long enough that, when I came to London, she decided to just give it to me since I would likely use it more.

Also, when I had first moved to London, I had bought one of the bigger, plastic carriers from the thrift store. I thought I was going to have to give Mum's carrier back, so I wanted one that was large enough to fit both hairballs if I needed to.

9 pm on the 3rd night of the new year. I heard the alarms, and grabbed for my phone thinking it was already morning. Not the case. I was shaken as I pulled myself from bed.

Do I respond to it, or has some asshole simply pulled the alarm for shits and giggles?

I decided I was not risking it, and quickly threw on my fluffy blue onsie. Honestly, it was the nearest clothing to me that I could get on. Aurora was frozen in place on the bedside table, which gave me time to go get the big carrier without worrying about her running under the bed. As I got the carrier, I flicked on the light to find Cleo.

She was crouched down behind my travel bag on my couch. I went over, and scooped her up. She didn't fight me until I was trying to shove her into the carrier. Once she was in, however, I had to grab Aurora. Trying to shove her in with Cleo didn't work. I had both of them pushing to get out because they were as terrified as I was.

I closed up the carrier once I had Cleo back into it. Then ran to the bathroom cupboard for the second.

The whole time, Aurora had slunk back to the bedside table. She remained there until I made to grab for her again. Then she tried to get to under the bed, but I already had her. I shoved her into the case, zipped it up, and threw on my jacket. In under five minutes, I was hauling it down the stairs to outside with a heavy carrier in each hand.

I know five minutes can be all the difference in an emergency situation. Still, my paranoid thoughts paid off. I didn't curl up and panic, wondering what I was going to do. How do I save my cats, and do I grab my laptop since it has my entire life's work on it?

Believe it or not, I left the laptop. And my phone, unintentionally, but the laptop I had known I was going to leave from contemplating it before. Things can be replaced, and most of the stuff on here can be re-written.

I'm going to have to rethink my plan on the carrier's placement, and how to react. After tonight, I'm almost certain when there is a real emergency, one of the two are going to end up under the bed.

As for why the alarm was pulled, I sort of got an answer. It was while I was waiting for my turn on the elevator back up, I noticed a woman to the side, crying. I knew her as a lady from the first floor. She had helped me out back in September when I didn't yet have my school bus pass, and needed to get to downtown to catch a train back to Chatham for the first time. She had given me a pair of tickets, and the timetable and map of the nearest bus, in exchange for five dollars.

This same woman had been mouthy with my mother during one visit regarding parking. Needless to say, Mum doesn't like her all that much.

The woman was speaking to a fire fighter when someone came up. She introduced herself with a handshake, and I heard her say, "It was my fire."

From my understanding, there had been a small fire in her apartment, which caused the alarm. Yet, it had been small enough that someone had already taken care of it before the first people had started leaving their apartments, let alone before the fire truck got there.

So, it technically had been a true emergency. Just one that had been handled before I even got out of bed.

Talk about a crazy night. I did find out who the cat people were. We and our friends in carriers were together by the dumpster, trying to figure out what happened. It was funny to listen to each of our stories about how we reacted to get our respective fur-balls.

Mine had been the easiest since they both froze where they were. The hardest was a pair of women with one cat. Theirs had hid himself away behind the shelves under the bed. This is why my bed-frame is elevated, and doesn't have anything underneath. Another anxious twitch from thinking about it too much. I was thinking I didn't want anything blocking if I need to grab one out of hiding for any reason.

Anyway, I have to be up for class that starts at 9 am. It's now 11 pm, and I'm finally starting to calm from the excitement. What a freaking night.

Mother Knows Best

My mother really knows how to bring out the worst in me.

It's the 8th, and I'm home from, yet another, four day visit to Chatham. It started after my Thursday class. Which was a really awesome class, by the way.

The professor, Marla, will be both my Painting 2 teacher, and Methods and Media teacher. Which means it will be easier to get in contact for questions and/or problems in either. I'm going to end up with 6 projects for the course of Methods, and all of them had to be under a theme.

After talking it out with my professor, and some inspiration from my friend, Maggie, my theme for the semester is going to be "Circus". It really should be called "fantasy". I think she didn't call it that because the entire class would pick it, if it was. Basically, I get to spend the semester drawing the very thing I already love to draw: dragons.

I've also gleefully discovered my classmates refer to me as the dragon girl.

Needless to say, I'm excited to get started.

That, however, is getting off topic. After Methods finished at noon, I came home, and got ready for what was supposed to be a two night stay with Mum. I was already heading downstairs with my things, as was normal, when it turned out my mother had come into the lobby. She apparently needed to use my bathroom.

Sad truth, my Mum has been in either of my apartments more times to use the bathroom, than to actually sit and visit. I kid you not. In the year and a half I lived on my own in Chatham, she had been in my place a total of 6 times. Four of which was because she needed to use the bathroom between clients, and my apartment was in between.

I'm certain she would have continued to do so, except I

was frustrated one of the mornings that she woke me up early, and wasn't even there to visit. She stopped coming over at all after that. At least until it was time for me to move to London.

With that in mind, it did not surprise me she wanted to come into my home for the sake of using the toilet.

I felt pretty comfortable with her coming in, for once. The only dirty laundry I had was currently in her van so that I could wash them at her house. My bathroom and bedroom had received full scrub downs. I had reorganized my bookshelf, got my Christmas stuff cleaned and packed, and had swept my floors. All within the week to two weeks I was home between Christmas and now. My home was a lot cleaner than it had been in some time.

I felt pretty proud of myself. Then, Mum waltzes into my apartment.

Right away she's at me about a smell. The source of which is a litter box that needs to be scrubbed rather than simply changed.

"Holy fuck, Anita. Is that litter box clean? You should do it now while I'm up here."

I was annoyed, but I did poop scoop. While in there, I realized I forgot the bag from cleaning out my crisper.

I had forgotten I had asparagus in there from who knows how long ago. Apparently, when it goes bad, it turns to mush in a bag. I figured that probably was part of the smell Mum was so worried about, and grabbed it to take out.

"Take this too," she grabbed a box of recyclables. She then proceeded to grab the empty cat food bag that was off to the side from when I opened the new one.

"And this," she snipped. But then she shook it, and looked inside. "Oh, you still have a couple of nuggets in here."

Instead of handing it to me so that I could pour the four morsels and the layer of crumb dust into the cats' dish, she proceeds to turn it over, and dump it on the floor. The floor I had actually swept the day before. Fucking nice...

I think she could tell she was pissing me off, because we headed out after that. Thankfully, it was cold out, so it helped cool my blood. It also helped that the recycle bins are at the back of the building, and Mum had parked out front. I had some time to take out my annoyance with strategically throwing each recyclables much harder than was necessary.

I reminded myself that she probably thinks she's helping. Yes, it is incredible rude to go into someone's home, and order them to clean the handful of things not done. At the same time, she's my mother. She probably sees it as coming into my bedroom and telling me to clean. Some tact would be nice, though.

Ask me why I have anxiety attacks about my mother coming into my home. I'm fully aware what is a mess, and what is not. I hate a dirty environment as much as she does, but there are days I just can't do anything about it.

Anyway, we make the hour and a half-ish drive to Chatham. The conversation was mostly what things are going on in Mum's world. There was a brief moment she was on me about my school registration, and figuring out OSAP. I mostly tuned out her criticism, and countered by telling her what I was doing to resolve the issue *myself*.

This is a side effect of asking her for money a little while ago.

Once in Chatham, Mum insists on playing that Pokemon Go app. During the drive around town to play, I asked about visiting my grandparents, and Uncle John and Aunt Sandra. It was decided I was going to stay until Sunday, instead. Since John and Sandra go over for dinner at my grandparents every weekend. It was just a matter of contacting them, and asking to have the dinner Saturday instead of Sunday.

Didn't end up happening. I was not informed so until Saturday afternoon, however.

It was only with my sister's intervention I even got to see them earlier today before leaving town. Mum had been putting it off every time I asked.

"We have all day tomorrow."

The next day would come, and I got the line again. And the next, except, on Saturday, it was "we'll see them tonight at grandma's."

Basically, Mum monopolized my time all weekend. I was in her house, having to ask permission to eat. Being sent to fetch things for her when she wanted them. I hooked her up with my netflix so that she could catch up on *Bones* the same as I had. It resulted in a marathon, which was a nice change up from playing Pokemon every minute of every day.

When being around her got to much, I spent most of my time working on a 1000 piece puzzle. Those things are my addiction, I swear. I'd say it was a good third to a half done by the time I came home.

If I wasn't at the puzzle, I was playing on my tablet, or sleeping. Needless to say, my independence annoyed Mum. She'd call me down to watch *Bones* with her, or to go play Pokemon, again. For a woman that goes on and on about how used to living alone she is, she sure demands company. It's kind of sad, which is why I made an effort to be around her as often as I could stand it.

This lead to the next piss off on Friday morning. My sister had text Mum to ask if she can go to that psychic, again, for her birthday. Seems fair to me, being it's her 23rd birthday. When we had gone, it was my 22nd. Plus, something like that was by appointment, so she couldn't exclude me with a last minute temper fit.

Except, the request set Mum off. I got to listen to her complaining all of Saturday about money. Sure, she tried to cover the complaining side of it as, "Oh, I was so careless with money this way" and "I have to learn how to live cheaply again". Add in another mention about my OSAP, and I got the feeling she was trying to guilt me for asking for $30. Even though I told her I would pay her back, and she's the one that said not to worry about it.

Mum also started to go on about how it was a good thing Cam had said something early enough for her to earn some extra cash to do it. I dared to ask if I was invited too. I figured it would be interesting to see if the lady said the same things, or if I had changed enough in over 3 years that she would 'predict' something different.

"Well, it depends on my hours between now and then," was her answer.

I hate the word 'depends'. Especially when my mother uses it. It's supposed to be a means of being hopeful, but I've learned enough that Mum is telling me "no".

"I don't think I'm even going to do it. It's so expensive," she covered. Then proceeded to explain for 20 minutes that it is pricy, and hinting at how I'm not included.

I didn't bother to mention I would have my own money by then, and could pay for myself. That would have opened up an excuse for Mum to be at me again about OSAP, or finding a job.

Like Saturday evening. I was already on edge. First, it didn't look like I was going to get to visit my extended family because Mum had put it off. Second, when Mum had sent me to get a pot pie from the freezer, she was flopping my phone around. Though there was nothing incriminating on it, I didn't want her going through my phone. Seriously, is a little respect towards privacy too much to ask? I couldn't snatch it away and take it with me, however, because that would look suspicious. The only option was to be quick to get the food. I was then quiet when coming back up stairs to see if she was snooping.

All that, plus hardly being allowed to talk without being interrupted, was getting to me. It got to the point that I just answer my mother with grunts, hmms, and huhs when she wants to be sure that I'm paying attention.

As we sat down to eat, I had been deep in thought about what sort of dragon I was going to draw first for our pencil medium. I decided I wanted to do a bipedal instead of a quadruped, which meant the wings would be it's arms and hands. I generally do Eastern or quadruped dragons, so I knew I was going to need a reference picture.

I asked Mum is I could use her printer for that very reason.

"You know what you should be doing," she said immediately after telling me it was fine. "You should be updating your resume. Then you can print some off."

I tried to hold my tongue, but after a few heartbeats of silence, I couldn't help but lowly hiss, "It was updated a month ago."

Which is was. While looking through my files when considering where to save this journal, I came upon an old copy. It was actually two or three versions old. It was easy enough to update. I'm not stupid. I know full well that I'm going to need a job. Especially by summer.

"I thought you couldn't find it," Mum countered my warning tone.

I explained to her that I had misplaced the usb with the most updated version, but how I discovered an old one lost in my documents.

She was quiet a moment, clearly thinking, and then, "Cam said you still have babysitting on it."

"Yes," I stated with another warning edge to my tone.

Cam had wanted to help me find a job before I had decided to go back to school. I figured it couldn't hurt. Thus, I let her see my resume. The one I had made through the local Goodwill career centre.

I wanted Mum to leave well enough alone. I'm not worrying about a job until March. Several of my counsellors had suggested it because I needed to make sure my current course load doesn't overwhelm me. Long and short, I need stability, and getting into a routine, before adding something else.

But since I had asked to borrow money from my mother...

"Well, I don't think babysitting is appropriate for an adult resume," Mum continued to press in a condescending tone.

In the same seething voice she had just used on me, I growled, "Well, the career centre people told me to put all job experience from the last ten years. I have babysat in the last ten years."

I was not meeting her eyes the entire time. I was also starting to be a little more rough with using my fork, and eating faster so that I could leave sooner. I have no doubt that my face was contorted into a scowl of some sort.

Luckily, Mum had already finished her food. "I still don't think it should be on there."

She went back to watching TV, and I hid away in the front room to work on the puzzle until 3 am. Long after Mum had gone to bed near midnight.

The entire time I was puzzling, I kept repeating inside, "She's worried, and she's just trying to help."

The damage was already done. The crueler inner voice was whispering again:

She doesn't think you can do anything for myself. Clearly, you're just useless and lazy, and a giant disappointment to her. You can't even make a proper resume. Even with a professional's help.

On and on I fought with myself. "I'm doing my best. She might not think it's good enough, but I can't fault myself for where I'm at. I'm making progress at my own rate, and I will be fine."

It took 2 hours of texting my sister before I was calm enough to go to bed. I didn't sleep, though. I lay awake, thinking about anything else I could. My novel, a new fanfiction, my drawing, or, after I put headphones on, just letting the lyrics wash over me. I was wide awake when Mum's older Chihuahua had been too noisy, and woke her before her alarm.

I debated for several minutes on just staying in bed. I was awake, though, so I figured I'd at least get some breakfast. Except Mum had finished the last of the milk, figuring I was going to be asleep until she got home at 9:30. There wasn't anything else, and I decided I was not going to ask permission to eat.

After she left for work, I had made myself a sandwich from leftover Swedish meatballs, shredded mozzarella, and two slices of rye bread. It was delicious. It was also satisfying because the previous night, I had asked if there were still meatballs, and she told me 'yes' but I was to have ice cream instead. Supper is in the oven, was her excuse. I knew I was hungry enough to have the meatballs, and still be able to eat later, but whatever.

I didn't want ice cream, though. My own little rebellion was that I grabbed an apple. Small enough to not spoil dinner, but solid enough that it actually took away my hunger pains.

I also want to put into perspective, it was around 7 pm, and we had not eaten since 10 am. Even then, it was a hash brown and bacon McMuff from McDonald's. Filling at the time, but easy enough to digest quickly and become hungry again. Mum doesn't eat often, and she doesn't like it when I ask to eat something between meals.

"I'm going to be making (Whatever mealtime we were at) soon," she'll say. On Saturday, when I had asked for something, she told me to go get the pie out of the deep freeze. Thus, the phone business.

As I said, that sandwich was extra satisfying. Especially after Mum's little episode this morning.

See, she had to leave for work at 6:30 am. Since I had nothing to eat, I went back to working on the puzzle, and just conversing with Mum about the day's plans. She went upstairs to get into the shower. Only to came out a moment later.

"I just remembered, I have those bags of cat litter in the back of my van."

That was from yesterday, because I had to be the one that put them in the van for her to begin with.

"Can you go get them for me?" Before I could say 'sure', she also said, "And if you want, there's also a bag of bird food back there that needs to be brought in." Then she went into the bathroom once more.

Maybe it was the lack of sleep. Maybe it was the fact I was already riled from the several other little things from this weekend. Likely, it was both, AND the fact that she had added "and if you want".

Thing about my mother's phrases, if she asks you to do something, but uses the phrase, "if you want", she's not asking. That's her cue that she wants it done now, or else she will throw one of her tantrums. As soon as she added that, the entire request changed from asking a favour, to making a demand.

I didn't feel like being a servant.

I stayed put, in front of the puzzle, contemplating a reasonable cover for why I decided I would do it later. I knew she was going to be pissed that I hadn't jumped when she told me to. She came out of the bathroom after finishing her shower, and didn't say a word, at first. Then she was overly cheery talking like normal again. I knew it was a false sense of security. I figured she thought I had got caught up in the puzzle, and just hadn't got to it yet.

Eventually, she came down to grab her coat. "So, are you going to get your coat on to come help me with that stuff?" The tone was cheery, again. As if it was just a simple request. It was the wording that was the warning. She expected me to get my coat on, and follow her outside, now.

"I figured I'd do it after when I bring my stuff out," I answered with the same false calm. "That way the door is opened less times."

"Well I'm already going out now."

"I'll do it later."

That's when the edge returned to her tone, "But it'll be forgotten later."

"No it won't."

"It'll get forgotten, and then I'll have to do it by myself with my bad back."

"It won't be forgotten because I have to put my stuff in the back anyway," I stated firmly. "It's easier to bring your stuff in the same time as I bring my stuff out."

She went quiet. I knew she didn't have an argument as to why it had to be done that very minute, other than, because she said so. If she played the angle that she's going to be driving around to clients with that stuff in her trunk, I was ready to counter with the fact she would have, anyway, because I would have normally been asleep at this hour.

She didn't argue it, though. Instead, she grabbed her things, and went out the door. I shouted out a excessively sweet "see you later", knowing full well it was going to irk her further.

Hey, if I'm going to piss off my mother, may as well go all in. It's not going to make a difference either way.

I was expecting her to slam the large door, but she didn't. She left it open. That's when I knew she was going to pull her, "I'll just do it myself" attitude. Sure enough, her and her bad back carried both 40 lbs bags inside, and the 10 lbs bag of bird food, in three trips. She didn't say a word, and I stayed where I was. I knew by this point, if I went to get the bags to take them into the basement-basement, she would have been on the attack.

I knew I had her wound enough she would have really let

me have it. Plus, I was in the mood to give as good as I got. There wasn't time for a shouting match before she had to be to work. Further more, I didn't want to risk pushing her too far, and having her hit me.

Now, my mother has never lost her temper enough on Cam or I that things turned physical. She never spanked us either. The only times I know of Mum hitting me was because of biting.

The first, Mum tells me, was when I was 2 years old. She says it was a reaction to the pain that she had not been expecting. Didn't help that I had done it from behind. At least that's how she tells it.

The other time was caught on camera. It was during one of Cam's birthdays. Mum was hiding a gift behind her, and I went to grab it. It resulted in us play wrestling, and, for whatever reason, I decided to bite to get free of her chock hold. My face was against her side. She let me go, immediately, and then gave me a hard slap across the face. In front of everyone. She was remorseful right after. It turns out I had drawn blood where I bit, so it wasn't a completely uncalled for reaction. Still, it's proof my mother can loose her temper enough to attack.

Heck, the fights between Cam and I are also proof that a temper can be driven in both of us. It takes a lot to get me to that point, but I was already part way there by that morning. I'm sure having Mum in my face would have lit the last of the fuse.

I suppose violence can be pulled out of anyone when pushed far enough.

Thus, the best thing I could have done was exactly what I did: stayed put.

I later text my sister, "I don't know if you still want to come with to London. Mum's in a mood, and I'm about ready to give her a long overdue piece of my mind if she starts on me."

I then went for an hour long nap. I felt better after I woke up, and Mum was fine by the time she got home. As it turns out, Cam had started texting her, and had got her mind focused on the trip to London. She also made it that she was at John and Sandra's house when Mum was to pick her up to leave. That's why I got to visit them, and the kidlets.

Also, since Cam was with us for the drive, I was able to curl up in the back to sleep while she kept Mum company up front. The drive home had been nothing to me, and they even stayed for a few minutes to eat poutine at my place.

Certainly a much more peaceful ending to a tough weekend. Boy, am I glad to be home, and going back to class in 6 hours.

Unexpected

I had an odd phone call from my mother earlier today. It was around 4:30 pm, just as I was getting ready to sleep.

"So, the people helping you at the school. You know, with your depression and stuff. What do you call them? I mean, what is their title? More than just a counsellor..."

Understanding what she meant, I answered, "It depends which one you're talking about. Linda is my personal counsellor. Anita is my academic counsellor. Dr Adams is a medical doctor..."

I was on edge. I thought maybe she hadn't let this weekend's events go, and was looking to discredit the people helping me again.

She picked up as quick as I trailed off, "Right. And what sort of things are they doing to help you?"

"Just talking through the issues. Meditation techniques. Ways to handle emotional moments better..."

Apparently, she had thought I said "Medication" instead of "Meditation". I had to correct her on that.

"So, they don't have you on any medication? Their not trying to push pills on you?"

By now, I was getting really confused. Not only was Mum admitting I had an issue, she wasn't trying to undermine it in any way.

"No, I told them when I first went in there that I didn't want to be put on medication."

Which I don't. I know my issues are situation combined with prolonged grudges, and self-isolation. Seriously, today I wanted to go home several times because I was worrying I wasn't interacting with my classmates properly. For some points, I felt like I was trying too hard. At other points, I felt like I wasn't involved enough. I ended up calming myself by building a clay dino-dragon creature.

When people asked why I was doing that when today was just a lecture day, I told them I was staving off boredom. It was enough to get me through, but I was exhausted by the time class was let out. I'm still tired now. Nick's texting had woke me up too soon, and I haven't gone back to sleep, yet. I suppose it was for the better, since I hadn't eaten before going to sleep. I'm letting my dinner settle before I attempt sleeping so I don't have more nightmares.

Back to the phone call with Mum.

It turns out the dog groomer and she had been talking. The groomer had asked how I was doing, and Mum had told her that I had been diagnosed with depression. According to my mother, the groomer said she wasn't surprised. She had seen it coming between our meetings, and the things Mum has told her about me.

It turns out the groomer had been suffering from depression for 25 years.

The point of all this is that the groomer had told my Mum of a homeopathic doctor in Woodstock. Which is 20 minutes from where I live.

"She told me that she suffered for years, and it took this guy's help to finally make a breakthrough," Mum explained in a tone akin to a sale's pitch. "She said that within a week, it felt like a weight had been lifted."

She told me when the next meeting is, how much it would cost, etc. Then she told me how, if this is something I wanted to try, she would be willing to pay, and drive me to the appointment.

Honestly, it was fascinating. My mother was not only accepting what I'm going through, she's trying to help.

I am curious. It sounds like this guy might have something that can alleviate the symptoms. Perhaps something to help my physical aliments, seeing as the only thing all these blood tests and shit are coming up with is 'your mental health is making you physically sick'. I don't know how much good it would do, if any at all. It would be nice to feel a little calmer, and less exhausted.

To be honest, over the last couple weeks I was actually starting to contemplate medication. I was thinking about Christmas, and my odd reaction to alcohol calming me. I'm really starting to wonder if, on top of the actual stresses, maybe there's some sort of chemical cause too. Maybe I just need to give it a try, and see if it does make a difference.

Yet, if this homeopathy method can help, I won't be stuck on pills the rest of my life. If it does nothing at all, then I still have counselling to help me through.

It doesn't seem like any harm. Except the fact that homeopathy is a pseudoscience, at best. I have an idea of what's inside most bottles of 'natural supplements', and it's not an encouraging picture.

The fact I'm actually considering this means I must be desperate. I think though, there is the touch of, "Mum suggested it, and it's the first time she's actually tried to help me concerning my mental health." I don't know.

What I do know is that I need to go back to bed. I'm already struggling to motivate myself to go to class tomorrow that I don't need 'lack of efficient sleep' on top of it.

A Waste

And... I missed class today. I was awake early enough to go, but couldn't get myself to leave my bed. No matter my self-affirmations, or self-encouraging pep talks, it wasn't until 11 am that I finally dragged myself out from my covers.

Even then, I told myself that if I was going to miss class, the least I should do is clean my apartment. I had the whole day to do so. You know what I ended up doing? I wiped down the glass panels in my coffee table, did less than a quarter of my dishes, and vacuumed a section of my main room floor. Which sounds like progress, but all of it took less than 30 minutes to do. Then I proceeded to go back to bed, and sleep until 11:30 pm.

What a waste of a day. And I feel like crap for it too.

I got up to attempt functioning a little today. Thus far, that entails eating a bowl of cereal, and watching random videos on youtube.

I wish this low spell would go away already. I have fun things to do, but no interest in doing any of them. I'm only doing this passage to feel like I've accomplished something. Even now, it just feels like I'm wasting time doing nothing.

This whole journal feels like a load of bullshit. In the end, it's just wasted time, and wasted space on my laptop. I'm just feeding this addiction of writing out my thoughts and feelings, but what is it going to amount to?

It's the same shit with school. Why am I trying? My sculpture teacher asked us to raise our hands if we hoped to get into a career involving the arts. I half raised mine because I do still want to be a writer. It just reaffirmed that I have no idea what I'm doing with my life. I have no plan. No hope. I just keep going through the motions, playing pretend.

I pretend I'll succeed in my courses. I pretend I'll finish my novel. I pretend I'll find someone that loves me for me, and raise a family together.

Except I feel like a failure to all of it.

I want to go back to bed. I shouldn't, because I've already slept so much today. But I want to. I suppose it's better than dwelling on all these negative thoughts.

Fidget

It seems the poor mood-set from the day before had bled over to yesterday morning. I had woken up around 4:30 am, and spent the time from there until 7:30 am fighting with myself to go to class. This time, it was because I was scared that I was going to 'fuck up my drawing'. I had already decided on Monday that I was going to add detailed scales to the dragon in my drawing.

Thing is, I usually avoid scales because I can't make them realistic looking. Since I was certain that I was going to ruin what I had done thus far by attempting scales, I didn't want to do it. Which resulted in not wanting to go to class at all.

Stupid reasoning, right?

In the end, I did get myself up, dressed, and out the door for the 8 o'clock bus. One hour earlier than class was to start. As it turns out, I was not the only one that had arrive to the studio excessively early.

The other person there was Maggie. I get along great with her. We had bonded over our shared love of Harry Potter. She is a vibrant, cheerful person that is still taming her own fire.

When I got into the class, and found Maggie, I was surprised. After chatting a little bit, we both had concluded that it didn't feel like it was going to be a good day. It was comforting to think someone else with sever anxiety was feeling off. That meant it wasn't me, but likely an environmental factor setting off everyone.

The funniest moment was after I had set my things out to start the day's work. Maggie was talking about possibly going to get a treat from Tim Horton's, but didn't know how bad the line would be. I told her I was considering going to pick up some candy from the variety store.

"Yes! Let me know when you are going, because I think I want to get some too," then in a more apologetic tone she added, "when you're ready though. I don't want to bother you from drawing."

I laughed, "I wanted to ask you earlier if you wanted to go with me, but I didn't want to bother you."

After we both laughed, we went to get our morning sweets. Then we came back to settle in for class. We only had until 11 am to draw because we were expecting a guest speaker. Turns out he was the old program coordinator, and he was there to discus video art. He seemed like a nice enough old man. A spirited 60 or 70 year old, with a large grin, and a Liverpool accent.

I've never done well just listening to lectures. I get distracted too easily, and zone out. I'm guessing it was a learned behaviour in order to zone out my mother when she gets into one of her fits.

Despite it's practicality in Mum's presence, it is not something you want to do during class lectures where it counts. In high school, I learned to manage by writing segments of my current novel. There were a couple of times I had a piece of clay in hand, and fidgeted with it, or simply doodled in my notebook. It kept me grounded, and meant I was paying far better attention. Except, to someone else, that was a sign of the opposite.

Needless to say, I had pissed off more than my fair share of strict teachers. Some of them thought they were catching me off guard by asking a question regarding their lecture. Only, I would be able to answer it. Most teachers let me be after that, seeing as I had proved I was paying attention. The exception was my first grade 12 teacher.

Yeah, I failed an academic level English class in grade twelve. Yet, I'm a writer.

Basically, all this adds up to the fact that I was continuing my drawing while our guest speaker was present. Naturally, half way through, he felt the need to stop and point me out. I guess he didn't see the times I would look up at the slides when it was relevant to what he was talking about.

"I concentrate better," I stated while meeting his eyes.

He didn't listen. He spoke over me as he continued, "Why are you drawing? Leave your work for later and enjoy."

"I concentrate better," I said again, more firmly. I could feel the eyes of the three combined classes that had come to see the presentation were on me. One of which is the current program coordinator, Gary. He intimidates the fuck out of me.

Honestly, he's a nice enough fellow; soft spoken, always trying to smile, and never has a harsh demeanour about him. It's his eyes, though. I hate looking him in the eyes because there's just something that unnerves me.

The guest continued to ignore what I was saying. I turned to face away from him since he was acting so childish when I was giving him an honest explanation.

"I'll put my light on you!" he finished in an joking tone. I could see the laser light he was using on the wall tracing me out. By then, I had had it.

I could feel my face lighting up beat red. I could hear snickers from some of those around. My blood pressure rose, and I had to leave before I started crying in front of everyone. Even after going through my thoughts to understand why I was crying, it didn't make sense to react that way.

At the same time, it does. I have a hard enough time feeling like I fit in with my classmates. This stranger just embarrassed me in front of all of them.

I intended to stay in the bathroom stall until 12:30 so that I could get my things cleaned up without having to face anyone. Class was supposed to be over at 12.

Yet, 10 minutes into my hour wait, Rachel, of all people, came into the bathroom.

"Annie, is that you?" she said in such a soft tone, I almost wondered if I had imagined it. I mean, I had thought Rachel was one of my classmates that didn't like me, or thought I was childish. We hardly talked, and when we did, I was the one beginning the conversations. I figured I was just an annoyance to her. I was greatly surprised that it was her that had sought me out.

    I don't remember answering her. I remember her talking to me, but not what she said. Eventually, though, I was coaxed out. She took one look at me, and opened her arms into a hug. I had clung to her as tight as I could for a few moments. Then I worried my tears would leave a wet spot on her lovely cream sweater, so I pulled away. I used grabbing a tissue, and blowing my nose as an excuse.

    She was there with me for a few minutes. Quietly encouraging me to come back. That "we want you back". I don't remember much else of what was said. I do know that any time I started to head back into being hysterical, she'd offer a hug. I'm pretty sure I had squeeze hugged her 3 or 4 times over the course of 10 minutes.

    She had to go back to class, and made it clear she wanted me to come to. She also understood that I needed a moment to clean up before I could return. I still went though. I couldn't tell you a word of the rest of the lecture because I was trying to not draw. It was beyond frustrating. I was only too happy when when he finished up.

    Another surprise happened while I was returning my drawing board to my locker. Devon, a girl from the A side of our split course, had come around to ask if I was alright. I realized she had been sitting next to the door when I got up to leave earlier. I had almost slipped thanks to my grip-less shoes, and she had been the one that had put out a hand to help me if I had fallen.

    Thing is, for someone of my size, I'm actually pretty good about regaining my balance fast. Practice, I guess, seeing as I'm a little klutz-y.

    I have to say that I am very thankful today is when my weekend officially starts. I even decided to have a giant cup of hot chocolate with my cereal this morning.

I think I'll try again on getting the place clean. I, at least, want to have my dishes completely finished, and the recyclables taken out. Hopefully today will be much better than yesterday was.

The Cardboard Cafe

I miss the Game Masters Emporium. There's walls of comics, boardgames, and figurines. The walls and ceilings have paintings from local artists. For example, the door to the back storage spot (and bathroom) is painted to resemble a tardis from the show *Dr Who*. I don't watch the show, but my sister is a huge fan.

The best part of it all is that you know exactly when the regulars will be in for what kind of event.

Enjoy Magic the Gathering? Wednesdays, Fridays, and the occasional weekend tournament.

Yu-gi-oh card player instead? Sundays.

My group was, of course, the board game players. We met as soon as the store opened at noon on Saturday, and played well until 4 or 5. Sometimes the games would even go until closing at 6.

It's easy to find people into the same hobby as you. I know for a fact that if you enjoy table top games, and walk in on Saturday, you'd be welcomed as if you'd been an old friend we haven't seen in forever (even if it's your first time). It's nothing to be a semi-regular, and get invited over to other regulars houses to continue playing after the store closes.

The games we play are greatly reliant on who brings what. Eric, of course, is always good about bringing his latest purchase to try out. He sayd he owns over 300 games. I thought I owned a fair number of games in my little cupboard.

The way the GME makes money from hosting Game's Day is that you buy from him while you are there. A can of pop, or some candy bars. If I had an income, I'd be ordering a number of board games from him that I have played with the Game's group.

All of this could just be a side effect of small town living. The regulars of one event tend to bleed over into the others, as well. We know who is who, and we generally all get along. There is one or two in the bunch that tends to be annoying... that's putting it nicely. We're open to new comers, but it's generally just us.

It's comfortable, and laid back. I can be competitive, and smack talk, and get the same treatment right back.

That wasn't the case here in London.

It's called the "Cardboard Cafe". The menu is delightful, and there's a giant selection of new and classic games for all ages along the one wall. I went as early as I could, thinking it would be like the GME, and fill up fast. I was deeply surprised to find there was me, the gentleman tending to the cafe area, and a young couple.

I thought maybe I was early. I went to search the games along side the couple, and offered a friendly hello. The girl was the friendlier of the pair, but not by much. I asked if they were regulars, and it turned out it was their first visit, as well. They then went back to observing the number of games to choose from, so I wandered around.

To clarify, I already felt horrible yesterday. I had gone too many days alone, locked up in my apartment. OSAP had finally come in, so I had a couple options. One was going back to the Saturday market, and seeing what groceries I can pick up. The other was finally seeing what the Cafe was about. It had been a long time since I last got to play a board game.

That's probably why it's good I haven't invested the amount of money I'd like into games. You need people to actually play them with. Otherwise they collect dust in the cupboard.

I had wandered around for about 10 minutes before going to talk to the gentleman behind the counter. I asked him when it was going to fill up with players. He said the rush hour was in the evening, but assured me there would be plenty of people through out the afternoon.

There was. All couples until about 2 pm. Then came a group of four that had a reservation, so I doubt they were open to a stranger playing with them, either. I left by that point. The only reason I got to play a game at all was because I had asked the first pair that I had initially met.

They were setting up their first game, *Jenga*, when I approached. "Do you mind if I play with you two?"

The guy looked at the girl, and she stared back. I knew that look. They were both urging the other to be the one to say 'no'.

"It's up to you," he said to her.

Her stare got a little harder.

"Or I can wait until more players come," I tried to sound aloof as I gave her an easy out. I suddenly wondered if I was intruding on a date, and should just go back to my lone table off to the side.

"Well, we'll need a third player for *Catan*," she finally answered. Her tone dripping with uncertainty.

"Okay," I tried to not sound too eager. I figured that this would be a chance to make new friends, and get a few rounds of games in. Either that, or it would pass the time until the regulars showed up, and I could play with them.

I patiently waited at my own table for them to finish their game of *Jenga*. It was easy enough to pass the time as I was enjoying my first ever Root Beer Float. A habit of buying from the business that was allowing us use of their space. Boy, was I happily surprised to learn it had ice cream in it!

I watched the comings and goings of a father with his young son. I was trying to not stare at the couple playing while waiting for whenever they decided to get to *Settlers of Catan*. What I did catch from them in their mild banter, and lovey grins just cemented the fact my presence was interrupting. I started to second guess playing anything with them, and just leaving to come back later during rush hour.

I was mulling it over when the blocks fell, and startled me. Then *Catan* was opened, and I figured there was no harm in one game. Better than going home, and feeling lonely again.

I ended up kicking ass. The boy, Ben, had never played before. The girl, Melissa, was good, but not as ruthless a player as my GME boys. I tried to be a good-natured, reassuring player since these two were nice enough to let me join. It took a lot to hold my tongue at points.

For one thing, one of the resource cards is called "lumber". Except it's just a picture of three stacked logs. Consistent players call it "lumber", but casual refer to it as "wood". Rule of thumb at the GME, though: if you leave an opening for a dirty joke, it will be pounced on. I had to force myself not to smirk every time we had to ask each other if someone "had wood" for trade.

Another thing is that when I started taking an early lead, they didn't team up on me to take me down. It made it easier for me to win, but it made it far less challenging then William and Eric would have made it for me.

The game was over pretty fast. By then, another couple had arrived and were playing their own game off in the corner by the window. Their posture, and volume indicated they were far friendlier people than the shy pair I was currently playing with. I figured I would go talk to them after this game, but I noticed that, while they were playing, once again they showed signs of being on a date.

I went back to the games wall, wondering if I should ask the pair I had already been talking to if they wanted to play a game I liked. I pointed a couple out to them, but they shrugged me off with one thing or another. I left them be after that.

Just as I started making another route around the store, another man and woman comes in. They looked to be in their thirties. Both were very good looking individuals, and well dressed. For some reason, I found them fairly intimidating. They had such kind smiles when I went to say hello that I grew more insecure. I tried to not look at either of them too long. I didn't want it to look like I was hitting on either of them.

I walked away from them pretty fast. Instead, I returned to the owner, and asked him about what time the regulars came in. I was hoping 4, because then I could wander downtown, and see what there was to see. He told me 7. So I went home, and figured I'd come back later.

I went to get a small box of groceries, instead.

The whole endeavour felt like a waste of time, and made me long for the GME. Oh, and it also turned out that to play with the games was $6 a person/day. Would have been nice if they had put up a sign somewhere explaining that. $6 for one half-assed game of *Catan*.

I was disappointed, and felt even more alone. All I could muster after that was a quick, microwavable lunch. Then, I went to bed at 3:30-4 pm. I got up once, at 2:30 am, but went back to sleep until 7 am.

It's now Sunday, and I have no idea what I'm going to do with myself until tomorrow. I'm sure Nick will want to make a stop in since we didn't meet up on Tuesday due to a snow storm. He'll be in St Thomas, tonight, so it's not an inconvenient drive for him.

I'm not looking for that kind of company, though.

I think I'm just going to curl back in bed for now. Maybe watch some movies, or work on my puzzle I really need to start making more friends. Or get a job to keep myself busy on weekends.

Just something so that I'm not alone all the time.

Escape Rooms and Candy Hugs

One idea can turn around a person's mood in a heartbeat.

Sunday morning I was still rather miserable. I didn't go back to sleep, but I didn't do more than work on my 1000 piece puzzle. My head was loud with self-loathing, boredom, and loneliness. I wanted to escape it, but I couldn't find an answer.

The cruel side of my inner voices started to play with me. Things like how I was only pretending to be a good artist. I'm going to fail this semester, and my academic probation will result in me not being able to take any college courses again for years to come. I'm going to fail this semester because I don't have what it takes to finish these assignments.

I'm such a disappointment to my family. And, "you know why someone as friendly and kind as you is always alone? Because you're weird, and childish. You have so many problems that no one want's to be around you. You're classmates are just being nice."

My mindset was in such a state that, for the first time I can ever recall, I was starting to worry for my life. I was questioning if I wanted to be alive.

I started texting people just for someone to talk to. Cam answered first, but her mood didn't seem to be any better than mine. The difference was, she was at work, and had a silent coworker nearby. She only wanted to talk about her stress and problems, and I tried to be supportive. I didn't know how to help, though.

I did get into a small fraction of what I was feeling. Not enough to overwhelm her, seeing as she already had her own problems. The conversation did not seem to be helping either of us, so it trailed off as our talks sometimes do.

I was alone again.

I told myself I needed to get out, and do something fun. I

knew Nick was going to want to hangout later. That would mean possibly going out for dinner, and then coming back to my apartment for the usual. I didn't have an interest in letting him work out his frustrations through my body, though.

I figured I could post-pone it, at least. See, last year my friend, Nelly, introduced me into something called "An Escape Room". It's literally a themed room that you have to put together the clues and riddles in order to undo the locks, and escape. All within the allotted time limit. Basically, a challenging game that was right up my alley.

Nelly was supposed to visit me in early to mid-October, and so we knew we were going to want to do an escape room. Turns out, London has two different escape venues. She and I go to the more involved one.

The other Escape Room place was clearly on a budget with it's decor. Still, it makes up for it with more interesting puzzles to solve. I managed to convince Nick to play with me in two of the two-man rooms sometime back. We did the beginner room, in order to get him used to how to play. We had so much fun that we ended up jumping into another room since it was not booked.

I decided that I really wanted to play an escape room on Sunday. Thing is, there are only so many two-man rooms.

I figured he would pass on the idea in favour of being at my place. I went back to considering telling him not to come at all. There were at least four or five times I had started writing a text. Another two attempts to write on my facebook, "does anyone in London want to do an escape room with me today?"

Needless to say, I didn't post either.

It was while my brain was calling me a coward that I grabbed for my phone, and texted Rochelle... Nick's mother.

I honestly adore Rochelle. She's a kind woman, and we can get into some incredibly deep conversation. She was probably the biggest help getting me through my break up with her own son. I think it helped to know that even his mother thought that him cheating was a dumb ass move.

The only thing is, I know she REALLY likes me being with Nick. Probably because I'm not afraid to call him on his crap when he's in one of his sour and/or judgemental moods. She's considered me one of the family since I was about 16-years-old. Heck, even when he and I were separated, she assured me that, no matter what, I was still like a daughter to her.

I've laughingly told Nick, "I think your mother ships us."

It does annoy him how close she and I are.

I text her, asking if she, and her boyfriend, would like to join Nick and I in doing an escape room. The four of us did end up going, and had a great time. The room was fairy themed, making it super exciting for Rochelle and me. We went for a sushi dinner, too, afterwards. It was super easy to get out of my terrible mood around them. Seriously, those three have a terrible habit of turning things into dirty jokes. Which is hilarious, but can be embarrassing.

There was a moment I tried to get in on the joking. Either Nick or Mark had said something about "you don't know Jack", or something along those lines.

The point is, Rochelle was being silly and said, "Who's Jack?"

"It could be your future grandson," I countered. I was referring to the fact that her daughter (Nick's older sister) is expecting her second child. I then realized I didn't know what she was having, so I asked, "Is she having a boy?"

Except Rochelle didn't hear that part. Her eyes were wide as she looked at me. The tell tale half-grin I see on Nick when he's trying to hold back joy- usually after he's told a terrible joke- was obviously inherited from his mother because it was there.

"You?" she chirped.

I was quick to correct the misunderstanding. It was a little unsettling to see her that excited of the prospect. She knows full well I'm not in love with Nick.

Like I have said, he is a friend. It's nice to have someone to debate movies with. This has been going on far too long as is, though. Rochelle's look reminded me that I'm playing with fire here. Where he would be heart-broken, at worst, continuing would cause rifts between members of my family, and I. His friendship is not worth that kind of damage to me.

Even so, Nick and I returned to my place fairly late. To my self-loathing, the sheets did end up shaking for us.

Still, the night had been so much fun that I was in a very good mood going to class yesterday. To make matters even better, I was getting along great with many of my classmates. From getting people with my corny jokes. Having in-depth conversations with Rachel. Hearing about Kennedy's trip she had just got back from.

Best of all, getting lots of hugs. You see, I had bought candy at the in-campus variety store. I had gone with Renee, but Maggie didn't want to come with. She looked a little down to me, so I bugged her about what kind of candy she would like. The bags are 3 for $5, it's really nothing. Eventually, I weeded out of her that she'd like some sour keys.

I proceeded to buy 6 bags of candy so that I would have plenty to share with my classmates. After giving the bag to Maggie, she tried to pay me back. Thing is, I know Maggie is a hugger too. That's why I told her that, if she really felt the need to pay me back, she could do so with a hug. I think that had cheered up her day as much as it had done for mine.

The same happened later with Renee. While I was buying the candy, she noticed one of the bags was gummy bears. She went on to say how this particular brand was her favourite because they included blue bears. Something that many other brands didn't have.

Since I was already sharing the candy, I gave her the gummy bears. She insisted she was only going to take a couple, and I laughed and told her to take half if she wanted. I had more than enough sweets to satisfy my addiction. I ended up not getting any of the bears myself, but Renee was beaming ear to ear. Well worth it.

She tried to give me money, and I told her, "same price as Maggie." Because, again, I knew she was a hugger. Probably even more of a hugger than me.

"Fine, I'll give you five hugs," she said. I only ended up getting one, but one is plenty.

I also got a hug saying goodbye to Kennedy for the day. It sounded to me like she had a lot on her plate for the evening, and I asked if her she wanted one. She gladly accepted. I also told her that if she was getting too stressed, she was to send me a message, and I would send her some jokes.

It was a good couple of days. I don't know how to express how happy I was to be making others happy through puzzle solving, dinner conversation, simple jokes, hugs, and candy.

I hope today will be fun, as well.

Courage

Saturday evening. It was late at night, and I was at my mother's for the weekend. Which went surprisingly well. There I was in the dark bedroom, listening to my Mum's light snoring in the next room over. I was trying to come up with a reason to deflect Nick's desire (expectation) to visit the following day. I was considering a lie to get him to back off regarding sex, but still hang around as a friend. I do, eventually, want to push him out completely, but I need him to know it's a choice, and not an angry retaliation.

His constant push about sex, however, needed to stop. Don't get me wrong, I've instigated a couple times as well. The more I'm around him, however, the more I'm reminded why I don't want him around.

Over tired from just functioning and visiting family, I wove one heck of a lie.

I told him that I would need to practice chastity for some time. The reasoning was that "my counsellor believes it's an addiction, and I need to let go of it for a while in order to focus on the root of the emotional state." I had to pretend I'm not allowed candy, either, but that just means I don't eat any in front of him. I told him I'm supposed to keep a journal of when I felt strong desires for candy or sex, to understand if what I'm feeling is a need to escape. Since "those are my vices".

Truthfully, sex is his vice, not mine. He believes it is, however, because I've yet to tell him a straight up 'no' when he starts sniffing about. I don't think he realizes that doesn't mean I'm saying 'yes'. It's more allowing things, and regretting before, during, and after giving him the opportunity.

He didn't take this sudden change well. When I told him he was still welcome to visit, his response was that he didn't believe WE would be able to keep our hands off one another. I know that's my own fault for letting him seduce me over and over. All for the sake of having company.

His logic was that he may as well not come visit at all.

I did feel terrible. I just wanted the sexual advances to stop, but still hang out. I even played his ego, "It means I'm trusting you to not try anything. Don't you trust yourself?"

"No," was his text back.

"Well, I'm glad you're at least being honest."

I did figure while I was coming up with the lie, to begin with, that I would allow one more time, and all visits after that were to be platonic. I'll give him credit for not immediately jumping at the chance. He was still 'sceptical' about us remaining platonic. I know it's just him trying to seed self-doubt in my head to weaken my resolve.

After the fairly long back and forth, we said our good nights. Nick was in a poor mood while I text him the next day after I got home. He did eventually come over, we watched a movie, and then went to bed. He didn't try anything until the next morning. After his alarm, at that, so I think he had purposefully put it earlier since I was "too tired" last night. It also gave the excuse to just have at it, and not get into the intimacy/play side of it. I detest quickies, but if that's how he wanted his last time with me, so be it. He clearly thinks he's going to have another chance.

Yesterday, however, I proved him wrong.

He had asked before leaving on Monday morning if I was up to company on Wednesday since he would be in town. I told him it would be fine.

The rest of Monday was great. I had gone to the school to view the show "Little Rays Reptiles". Which was super cool. I got to hold a tarantula for the first time. I adore all animals, but there are just some I know better than to touch and handle. Big spiders being among that list of "admire from afar" since I have no idea which are deadly, and which are harmless.

The handler was letting people hold it for pictures,

though, so clearly it was not the dangerous sort. I gave it a go, and I've very happy I did. It felt like someone was softly touching my palm with pipe cleaners. I had been told that tarantulas feel weightless some time before, but I was still incredibly surprised by it.

I would have missed that if I had stayed locked up in my apartment all day, like my first intention. Of course, writing that I'm thinking, "if I went to the school, why the fuck didn't I just go to class?!" I probably wouldn't have missed Tuesday, or felt like shit on Wednesday if I had just gone.

I did tell Linda about my lie to Nick. She thought it was hilarious. "I don't mind. Honesty is the better quality, but, in this case, you should use whatever lie you can to separate yourself from scenarios you are not comfortable with."

That helped me feel less guilty about lying instead of just doing the brave thing, and telling him off. Funny thing is, I've heard the word "courage" and "brave" directed at me a couple times the last two weeks.

Once for being "brave" by going up to introduce myself to new people at the Cardboard Cafe.

Several times for holding the spider. The exception being my mother. She hates spiders to the point that videos or pictures freak her out. Naturally, she was the first person I sent a picture of me holding the tarantula to.

The other time was Wednesday. It was definitely a low day. Most of the morning and afternoon was spent in the throngs of a crying fit in my bed. I tried to distract myself through playing video games.

I took a break between my gaming, but just to see if anyone was available to chat on Facebook. There were a couple people online, but I didn't reach out because I felt like I'd be bother them. Plus I knew to expect Nick in the evening.

My sister did leave a crap tone of videos in messages to me, though. They did help.

In my browsing, I came to learn January 25th was the day Bell was doing something called, "Let's talk". I don't know what it was other than something that was raising money for mental health. There was a conspiracy that it was a money grab. I don't know, but several friends with mental health were sharing their stories because of it. Or leaving comments about raising awareness for mental health. So, I wrote the following message on my status:

I didn't realize today was about talking about mental health to raise awareness. So, little late in the day, but here it goes.
I suffer from clinical depression, and sever anxiety. Some days, I can't leave my bed, let alone my home, because I would rather sleep than deal with my own thoughts. I worry about everything (my looks, my attitude, what I say...), but a lot of the times, I have no energy to fix it.
I can be told 1000 compliments, and only hear the one negative thing. Or worse, mentally twist them until they are all negative, or I'm convinced they are lies.
I will cry because my brain has convinced me I am a failure, a disappointment, and/or that I'm unloved.
I doubt myself to the extent I am constantly seeking advice or affirmation, because I don't trust any little positive thought I have of myself. If I'm asked to repeat myself, I change the wording.
I feel like I have to say smart things, or else I feel dumb.
I feel like I have to do kind things, or give compliments, to compensate for people having to put up with me.
I've been working on this message since 4:30 pm, but I keep deleting it because admitting what's going on makes me feel weak and worthless, and my head tells me that people are just going to hate me or feel sorry for me.
Even while I'm writing this, I am telling myself "it's not that bad. I'm probably making it sound worse than it is." But the problem is, it is that bad. Unfortunately, it's not talk about enough, or treated as a serious issue.

It was hard to leave that where my family could see it. Mostly my mother. Surprisingly, she didn't message or call me to ask why I put that up, or tell me I'm over acting or attention seeking.

She just left a comment, "Hugs baby you got this!"

It's still odd having her not trying to deny or undermine my problems. I'm a little paranoid that this might be a phase, or an act. I'm sure that's just me and my trust issues again.

Her's wasn't the only comment, but it's the only one I truly paid any attention to. I know Aunt Sandra had put in their comment that I was being courageous for sharing my story.

The point is, I have been told I'm a brave person. A lot of times, I can agree to the statement. It's because I grew up either taught or told that "true courage is admitting your scared, and doing what needs to be done regardless". I'd never make friends if I let fear and distrust keep me from reaching out to meet new people. I'd miss out on a lot of experience, like riding a roller coaster or singing karaoke, if I didn't try.

Sometimes fear or insecurity wins, but I can only do my best, right?

It's why I grin from ear to ear as I tell people I'm a bloody coward. I know they will think otherwise when I go out and do something exciting, or unnerving. I know, however, that I'm terrified beneath it all. I still say it, though, since admitting it is how I become a braver person.

Talk about being a walking paradox.

The lie may not have been courageous, but I had enough strength to hold my ground on Wednesday.

He still tried to convince me without openly saying it was what he wanted. It's not a new tactic. It was one he developed during the many other time I've told him I wanted the sex to stop. He starts by waiting for me to show interest, or to out right instigate.

He doesn't realize that, sometimes, I start poke fights to be annoying. Not to instigate touch.

When I don't show any sexual interest, he gets touchy, and even makes sure I feel it pressed against my back when trying to sleep. It's why I think he pretends to be a lot more tired than he actually is when he comes to visit. There have been a few too many times that he's "so tired" that he's dozing on my couch, but suddenly alert when it's time for bed.

I have tried detouring this by having him on the couch, but that didn't last. Again, this is a process. When I finally decided it was bed time Wednesday night, he was allowed to sleep in my bed with me. He pretended he was showing resolve by keeping his boxers on. But he was still being touchy.

I just accepted the eventual massage, and pretended it put me to sleep. The next morning, I was actually tired. I barely moved when his alarm went off. I actually went back to sleep, which clearly frustrated him.

His alarm is for 5 because he has to be to work for 6:30 am. It's a half hour drive, but he doesn't wake with the first alarm. Plus I think he stops home before heading into work. That's why, normally he's up and out the door by about half past 5, or quarter to 6.

He conveniently had "accidentally" turned off his alarm instead of hitting snooze that morning. He was still awake by 6, though. He had an "oh well" attitude, and said he just wanted to stay and snuggle. That's why all he got was snuggles, and I ignored his 'waging tail', as I call it.

Funny secret: I say it to his face, but when I refer to it as a 'waging tail', it's a veiled insult. I'm calling him a 'horn dog'. That may not seem like an insult, but that's me insinuating he's a hormone driven bastard. If people that I've called 'horn dogs' knew that's what I meant, I'd probably be in some serious shit. But, he thinks it's a joke.

When it became clear he didn't intend to just leave, I said my alarm was to be set for 7 so that I could shower before school. I figured he would get the hint that that was when I wanted him to leave by.

He didn't.

When my alarm went off, and he started to 'snuggle' some more, I yawned and told him to just shut it off. I turned over, and, once again, ignored him. It was 11 by the time I could no longer sleep. Which worked perfect because I had an appointment for noon. I had a reason to get up, shower, and kick his ass out. I just made the mistake of mentioning being glad it was only an hour so that I could come home, and go back to bed. He had ended up waiting for me to finish my appointment.

Before that, however, he seemed to have got the hint that just being a little touchy wasn't peeking my interest. He couldn't push, because then he risked pissing me off. I caught the pensive look on his face more than a couple times Thursday morning. He had to make it seem like my idea, or he wouldn't have an argument against me telling him not to come back.

Thing is, he's not as clever as he thinks he is. Teenaged me may not have noticed the manipulative side of him, but adult me is a paranoid asshole without a drop of trust for him.

As I'm stretching, and gaining motivation to shower, he once again makes his tail obvious. Even going so far as to cause it to wag so that I'd notice it. Then he suddenly backs off, "Sorry."

I shrug, "it's natural."

He's then quiet for a couple minutes, and then, "You know I really can't help looking at you. You know, like this. It's not the same with clothes on. I'm not sure what it is."

I mentally roll my eyes. I wanted to say, "you just like looking at a half naked woman that you think you're going to get some from." I stayed quiet though.

He continues to try to sweet talk. "Maybe I just like

seeing your..."

I almost laugh out loud now. He was trying too hard that he didn't have a genuine compliment lied up that wouldn't make him sound like a horn dog.

"Curves?" I supply. I was hoping he would say it, just so I could tell him, "down boy". I definitely had my inner bitch dial to 11.

He didn't bite, though. "Maybe," he tried to smooth over. "I think I like seeing your skin."

This did cause me to snicker a little. I attempt to cover with a silly, "It's the freckles." I hold up my arm to add to my point. "I'm practically a dalmatian."

He didn't respond, but he did rub his hand on my hip. "I think it's because it's so smooth. And soft."

I move away, using the need to get up to stretch as my excuse. "So, you like young girls with firm skin, eh?" I used a joking tone to hide the fact I was implying he was shallow.

I don't remember his exact wording, but it was back to him talking about how frustrating this dry spell is going to be. He comes up to hug me from behind as I'm gathering my clothes for the day.

"I know I can't in, but maybe on?" His tone is joking, but the words piss me off.

"I'm sure you'll figure something out," I shrug him away. As I'm leaving the room, I can't resist tossing over my shoulder, "There's klneex on the dresser. Try not to make a mess of my sheets, okay?"

I suppose that's the nicest way I could tell him to fuck himself. Either way, I was quiet pleased with myself while I showered.

Of course, he wasn't finished. He decide that after the water for the shower started would be a good time to use the toilet. I told him to go ahead. I kept my back to the wall so that I could see either side of the curtain in case he decided he was going to peep. He didn't.

I listened for him to close the toilet lid. Once he did, I waited for the sound of the door's bottom swishing against the tile to signal he left. Except, he lingered. The lack of shadow on the curtain, however, meant he was near the door. It's a small, bathroom after all.

He stayed just long enough for me to start getting annoyed. I was starting to wonder if he took my Klneex idea as permission to masturbate near me. That would have had some amount of sound to it, though, so I don't believe that's what he did. Besides, he would have made sure I knew that's what he was doing.

Gratefully, that was the last of his up-front attempts. I went to my appointment, told Linda about my lie, and also discuses the possibility of volunteering at the Children's Museum. I have no idea how much I'd be able to concentrate on the job in there, though with my woman-child heart.

After my appointment, Nick and I came back to my place. We played video games for a few hours. Then I cooked dinner, and we watched the *Goosebumps* movie. This lead to conversation about various *Goosebumps* books, which reminded me of the show. He mentions the show is on Netflix, so I go and search for certain episodes.

This leads to more nostalgic viewing, and Nick getting tired. He ended up curling up to sleep with his head on my arm. Which was over my lap because I wasn't letting him get too cozy, again. I had told him before heading for my appointment that he was welcome to continue visiting, but he wasn't staying over for another sleep over.

It was about eleven when he apologized for, once again, dozing off.

"That's okay. I was going to leave you be, and kick you out at midnight." Because his presence so late was starting to bother me. I knew he might use how late it was, and how early he had to be up as a reason to ask to stay.

He nodded, "do you mind if I just go have a quick nap then?"

"Go ahead." I was stuck on watching 90s *Goosebumps* episodes.

I had also been texting my sister some cringe worthy quotes from the show to laugh with her over. She eventually got tired of texting, and just called. We ended up chatting for a little over an hour. I wasn't worried about being quiet about it, because it was after midnight. Nick needed to wake up, and get out. I actually had a great time talking with Cam.

It left me in a good enough mood to have some patience with him when I went in to officially wake him. The first time, I curled up next to him, and started poking his side. He said he was awake, so I left the room to finish the episode that Cam had interrupted when she had called. There was only 5 minutes left on it, after all.

Once it was finish, and he still hadn't emerged from my room, I went back in. This time, I switched on the light, and removed the blankets. He mumbled that he was awake, again, and said he had known I was coming. He even started talking to me about some of the things he had overheard me discussing with Cam. I said "okay", turned the light back out, and decided one more episode.

It was about 5-10 minutes in that I realized I still hadn't heard him getting up. By then, I was still in a semi-good mood. I decided it was time that I turned full pest. I turned on the light again, opened the window to let the cold air bother him, and even smacked him with a pillow. A really hard one to the side of his head because he thought he'd just cover his head with one of my other pillows. By that point, the play was out of me.

I left the light on, and left the room again.

I finished the episode, and he *still* had not rose. I was silently seething by then. Did he think if he played up how tired he was that I would take pity on him?

I walked in, and stood at the foot of the bed. He had that slightly heavy breathing people get when they're not quiet asleep enough to be snoring. Yet, still definitely asleep. I stood there a good minute just to prove the point that he didn't know I was there. Thus, he could not just say again that "he was awake".

I didn't touch him. I didn't yell. I just spoke with a low warning, "You know, I'd like to go to bed."

His eyes popped open, and he met my gaze. "Sorry," he muttered. Same as he had the last couple times. This time, he stretched. I left the room to avoid smacking him again, with something harder than a pillow. It was almost 2 am when he finally left. In the end though, he left, and didn't get what he had wanted.

Needless to say, I woke up quiet refreshed this morning. I also went to the store and bought several bags of candy to enjoy as celebration. I know it's going to take all the courage inside me to continue, but it was one step closer to the right direction.

Re-freed

I've taken another step towards fully ending it with Nick.

Last night while we texting one another, the topic about one of my other exes came up. Nick does know about them. When he had learned during that year his new girlfriend was pregnant that I had slept with two different guys (in the course of a year, mind you), he had sneered.

He added insult to injury that he and I definitely could not work it out now, because I was "unclean". I still bring that up when I'm feeling particularly vicious towards him.

As for the exes, I have talked to Nick about why, of my opinion, they didn't work out. As we were talking, however, it became clear he was mixing up which problem had been faced by which relationship. Shouldn't be that hard. I've only dated 4 other men than him. One of which I didn't even have sex with.

In a moment of going in circles, and his teasing my choice in men, I wrote, "I don't have a good track record, okay :P"

We glazed over the comment. His attention was turning the conversation to how frustrating having to practice self-control is. He was more interested in trying to get me thinking about it through rather graphic descriptions of what we're missing out on.

I side stepped each description with a joke, because I knew it annoyed him. I didn't get into our usual "first to break" game. It would have encouraged him to continue his descriptions, and think that I was going to give in on his next visit. My lack of interest eventually got to him.

"Ya, but it's so much fun… Unless… Do you feel bad on the inside later? Am i part of your bad track record that you feel trapped like with Jared and Ian? That you know you shouldn't but you still choose to because your getting attention."

That message came in at ten to midnight. My stomach

twisted because I didn't want to lie. The thing is, agreeing to how he said it, no matter how true, was just cruel. I tried to tell the truth with as soft a blow as I could:

"You want the honest truth? Yes. I like being friends with you. I like going out and doing friend things with you. And there are times for sex that we are rocking it, and it's safe because it's just sex.

But there is a lot of times you want more. Where you crowd or where we have sex because it makes You feel good. I've been really trying to be considerate of you but this is a roller coaster. I can't just fix the hurt, betrayal, and distrust in only a few short years.

"I still look for manipulation. You say things that makes me realize you think this is more than fwb (FWB+ as you put it)

"But there's moments when you're trying to be intimate about us. About a month ago there was the conversation where you said you don't need a service, you decide when you're married, and I got spooked. I thought, 'does he think I'm his wife?'"

His message was next, "You agreed when I said that though... I feel there's too much history that plays a factor... but ok..."

Or conversation carried on for two hours. By the end of it, he had unknowingly admitted that he was using me for sex. I had cornered his responses in such a way that he had no choice but to admit he was interested in another girl. I told him that I don't care if he's interested, and fully support him going for it. If he's starting to make advances, though, then we are to be friends, only. Anything else would be "treating me like side ass".

He kept arguing that he had been looking only. That, "if thinking it was the problem, he's been treating me like side ass for a long time".

The comment had stung, but it also strengthened my cause. I'm done letting him use my body. I'm done with his little games. I made it clear to him that it was not thinking that was the problem. It was the fact that he had openly said he was making advances to another woman, but only joking ones.

He played up that he only really started looking this past week. As if to unofficially blame me for his lack of hormone control. I called him out on it. I told him that I would still welcome his company, but sex was out of the equation. I also told him that I wanted to do a month of just text friends.

I told him that it was to allow me time to think clearly, and work through my problems with my counsellor.

The truth is, I just don't want him around. He was already on the verge of a temper tantrum when I told him I wanted friendship only.

"Not surprised though... I did think the other day that things were nice. That i can hold this for a while. As soon as I thought it I was scared. Whenever I have that thought, something changes and makes thing hard again... Just didn't expect it to be you... After having reached a comfortable balance with you..."

He kept up that for a while. Poor him. Why is life always so hard? Why can't things just work out?

I know the play. He's done it to me before. It's what got me into this mess of being involved with him after she had left with their kid to begin with. It started because I was trying to comfort him. I never got my closure after our break up all those years ago. There was still a part of me that even loved him.

It was only after we interacting again that I saw him for who he really was. I had been trying to push him away for over a year. The problem is, I was trying to do so in a way that didn't hurt him. I don't think it's out of love, because I'm old enough now to realize what I loved was the man he has the potential to be. Not the one he has chooses to be.

He sees nothing wrong with himself, and blames fate for every time something goes wrong in his life. Yeah, sometimes fate can be a dick. A lot of times, though, it's because you make the choices that fuck you up.

I can admit I've made a lot of bad choices. I just take it as a reminder that I am human. I'm prone to make mistakes, and I have to live with them. Allowing Nick back into my life being one of them.

But you know, I don't regret it. I no longer wonder if things would work out between us. I no longer think that, if I had given him the chance back then, would he have picked me over her? I know now that, if we had tried again, I never would have seen who he really is. He would have had me wrapped around his finger, fooling around with other women behind my back, and I probably would not be allowed to experience life the way I'm meant to.

True, my mental health causes me to doubt, and even loath who I am. There are also days I am strong enough to shrug and say, "my journey isn't over." Maybe I just feel great today because I know I'm getting my life back on track. I have taken away his control over me. As terrifying as it is, a part of me whispers, "there is better out there."

I had my cry early this morning. I don't why. There could be that teenaged me dying inside that still wants to save him from his own misery. Maybe it was because I'm scared that I'll let him back in when loneliness gets too much again.

But you know what? When I woke up this morning, there was a small bit of lightness inside me. Not a lot because self-doubt wants to overshadow it, but it's there. It reminds me of when I'm hiking in the woods, or singing my lungs out. A sort of excitement about possibilities.

I don't think there is an official term for the saying. Maybe "hopeful" would work, but not really. It's more like a combination of 'relieved' and 'free'.

"Refreed"? Actually, let's add a hyphen and call it, "Re-freed".

You know what, I'm calling it that. That's going to be my writer's contribution to society.

REFREED: an adjective describing the euphoric sensation that happens after overcoming a long time struggle. Especially if that situation and/or person directly affects one's self-esteem.

You know, by putting it that way, I could say I had been "re-freed" when I admitted to "Dog-girl".

I'm laughing right now, for the record. I'm imagining the look on people's faces if I were to actually use that in conversation. I'm not sure who would be funnier: my mother or my sister.

Probably Cam. Depending on her mood when I say it, she'll likely come out with some funny comeback, or, you know, just say I'm weird. But I say, embrace the weird!

I also say that I am over tired, and should consider laying off the sugared drinks for a while. Especially dark colas (cough-root beer- cough) since I'm fairly certain those are caffeinated. That, or I'm so "re-freed" that I'm starting to get giddy.

Today, I am happy.

Weakness

I feel empty today. A stark contrast to my last passage, I know.

It's 4 am on Monday morning. My sleep is backwards that I likely won't be tired until 8 or 9. It's because all I have been doing for days is sleep. Nearly all of last week was spent in my bed. I know I left myself too vulnerable emotionally by shutting myself in.

Sure enough, when Nick text me on Wednesday to chat, it opened the door for him to come over Thursday. Things happened that I regret happening. He then had to go to a meeting with his ex to discus custody and such on Friday.

Of course, I was not aware that was the meeting he was talking about. Not until he text after finishing up to ask if he could stay another night. I allowed it, though I probably should not have. It was just nice to have someone to talk to.

Thankfully, I was much more resilient to his advances the second night.

I haven't text him since, and he seems to be leaving me alone for a little while. Probably only until next weekend when his hormones will cause him to sniff around. I don't plan on talking to him.

I said that last Sunday, though, and look how that turned out.

Just like how I said I would spend the weekend catching up on my classes. I had even went to class Thursday to talk to my Painting/ Methods and Media professor to know what to catch up on.

I didn't keep to that plan, either.

Painting starts in only a couple hours, and I don't want to go. How do you explain to someone that you didn't spend the weekend catching up because you were confide to your bed, even though you perfectly health? It feels like I'm just being lazy, and procrastinating. I'm just coming up with excuses for not doing things, again.

    I was actually starting to catch up on some of my chores too. Not long ago I had sent a text to my sister joking about how you can actually see my counter. Once again, it's disappeared beneath dirty dishes, and trash inside groceries bags since I already have a large garbage bag full, and haven't taken it out, yet.

    At least I've remembered to keep on top of my personal hygiene. Only because laying in a bubble bath was a step up from laying in my bed.

    Which is why I'm writing this tonight.

    My lack of productive activity, combined with overwhelming loneliness, and probably a fair helping of regret lingering in there, have all team up with the crueler side of my thoughts. This is the second time in as many months that I have actually started to fear my train of thought. I know this is not the first time that hope seems to slip away, and I'm left wondering, "why am I bothering?"

    The thing is, when this self doubt would pop up, I had accomplishments to counter them. I had dreams to cling to, and wipe away the tears.

    As I cried tonight, I couldn't think of reasons to live. Every time I told myself a reason, it would be burned to ashes in seconds. It's a good way to give yourself a headache; that's for sure. I'm terrified of myself right now. I feel like I have considered what ways would cause the least painful death, while also making it look like an accident to make it easier on my family, far too many times.

    Let's be honest, once is too many times.

    I think of my dreams. They feel rainbow framed, never to see reality.

    I can't hold a job. I can't even stick with school in a program I should be excelling in. I can't be responsible enough to fucking take out the trash like a regular adult.

I thought of my family. First my imaginary future one. It's a bitter-sweet thought to believe that, maybe someday, I could find love. Someone that actually gives a shit about me. Who can see how hard I'm working on the inside to be better than I am now. Not use me, and then leave me to wallow in my mental hell.

Naturally, I think of children, too. Sometimes I am realistic, and think that I'll have 2 or 3. Sometimes I'm a little more ambitious, and imagine rearing an entire baseball team. There is a sad part of me, however, that knows any possible children I have would have to be from my future husband's previous relationship, or adopted. But really, with my mental health, I doubt any father's would want me to be a step-mother to their children, and any adoption agency would turn me away in a heartbeat.

I also thought of my real family. I always think of them during the down swing of this horrible pendulum. My mother and sister are at the forefront of those thoughts. Tonight I seemed to tempt fate when I thought, "They already live their lives without me. They only text me once in a while. I know I worry them. Maybe it would be easier if I disappeared. They wouldn't have to worry about me anymore."

Then I remembered a talk Cam and I had a week or two ago. One of her co-worker's had a death in the family.

"I couldn't imagine loosing my sister," she had text. I cried then, as I am crying now. In her own way, she's telling me to hang in there.

I think of Mum, and how she gave up so much for us. She chose to have me, and raise me. Taking all that time, effort, and love, and saying, "I'd rather be dead" just feels wrong.

Despite our rocky relationships, they inspire some amount of fight in me. It triggers this more wild, more instinctual side of me. It's the side of me that wants to live, and will fight to survive. I don't like dealing with that side often because it makes me restless, and quick to aggression, but I need it. Just until I get my footing again. I want to try for them.

February 14th

Thursday snuck up on me this week. I find it hard to believe it's already the 9th of February.

That also means one of my least favourite days of the year is coming up. I may be a romantic, but I am no fond of February 14th. It's not a problem with Valentine's Day, it's just February 14th seems to be unlucky for me. Or it's an easy date to remember when things happen because it's also Valentine's Day. I'm not sure.

The first was the year I turned 19. Along with all the other lovely traumas of that year, it was also the year Nick and I wanted to have a family. When I hadn't had a period since mid-December, we were edgy, yet excited. More terrified than anything, but that's because we were still very young, and I was planning to go to college for Nursing.

All the tests were negative. As another day stacked up, the more he and I talked about family, and the more hope started to overtake my nerves. We had been contemplating coming clean to his mother, despite the negative tests. I had never gone so long without before. Only, the morning of the 14th, I woke in Nick's bed with sheets soaked in blood. It was the first time I got the truly bitter taste of hope being swiped out from under me.

Don't get me wrong, I have been disappointed many times in my life. What I felt that day was different. It was like having a dream about being at a feast, only to wake up and realize you're starving. For some time, I had convinced myself that I must have been expecting, and just miscarried. I was too frightened to accept the alternative.

I know better now that there is a very good chance I'm infertile. It was the first time I had experienced the real possibility that I may be incapable of having children. True, it was not as scary a possibility then as it is now that I am getting older. It still sucks, and I always have Valentine's Day to remember that.

Skip ahead to that October, Nick had left a rose and card for me on the fence. I thought he was apologizing, and opened myself to talking to him again. That's when he dropped the bombshell that the other woman was pregnant. In the same breath, he sorrowfully groaned that, "she doesn't even want it."

Needless to say, that statement had hurt me worst of all. Again, at the time, I had convinced myself that I had lost a baby only a few months prior. Not only had she 'stolen' my boyfriend, but she was pregnant with his kid, and didn't even want it. I remember thinking, "how can anyone be so selfish?"

I knew he wanted to be a father. I also knew that he wanted a family unit with both parents present in a child's life. I figured that, if she truly did not want the baby, Nick and I could get back together, and we would raise it. I had posed this idea to him, and he disagreed. At first it was, "she might not agree".

That's what lead to me sending HER a message. I had been confused by her response. At the time, I had believed she must have realized the kid was key to holding onto Nick. After some cyber investigation (I was 19, don't judge me), and some time for me to grow up, I have come to realize she probably never said she didn't want the baby. She probably had said something along the lines of being uncertain, and he had twisted her words. Then, knowing my desire for a family, he used that to get me to hook me back towards him.

I'm still miffed to think that it had worked. From the moment he told me until February. He would say a problem he was having with her, and I would bring up again that I was there. He would counter that he didn't want a split family. There's a long back story behind his logic that a warring household with both parents is better than the parents being separated. It's not my story to tell, though. When he talks about it, he's still incredibly bitter.

With February in full swing, I was getting annoyed. I was basically told that my years of love and loyalty meant nothing to some woman he wasn't happy with, but will stick with because she could have his child, and I couldn't. I decided that I was going to fight fire with fire.

It was freezing cold night. I don't know if it was the 14th, but it was close enough. We sat in his truck after playing Yu-gi-oh cards at the GME on Sunday. Mum thought I was at Ben's place, since that's where we usually all went together to continue playing after the store closed. When Nick still would not listen to me, I decided to seduce him.

The logic was that I could entice him with sex. And, if I fell pregnant, he would be free to choose because either way, he would be leaving one of us as a 'split family'. Needless to say, that had been a dark time of my life, and I am quit ashamed of my actions.

Getting his attention was not hard. He said that she had not wanted to have sex since learning she was pregnant. Which means it had been a couple of months for him. Believe me, he starts sniffing around for release after a week. I even preformed oral for the first time.

It was something he had been hinting towards for a long time, but that I refused to do when we were younger. I still detest the action to this day.

After I had made him feel better, he seemed to grow a conscience, and did not want to go any farther.

I told him I would do it again the following Sunday. He was all for it. Yet, as the week continued, I was overcome with guilt, and self-loathing. I realized that I was now the side chick, and that was not right. It was either Tuesday or Wednesday before I finally sent her a message that was both an apology, and a warning that he was still a cheater.

I pulled away from him after that. Still there enough to keep tabs on him, and get pulled into his drama every few months. After that, though, I had finally started dating other guys. Ian was more than happy to jump in as rebound. Honestly, he's a horn-dog too, he's just actually loyal to any girlfriend he's with.

In the grand scheme of things, that was a bitter-sweet 14th. I think that was when I finally learned that Nick would never be loyal, nor would he love me as I deserve. Granted, that is a lesson that took getting involved with him again before it sunk in, but everything is a process.

As for the year after that, I wish I could say it was Nick-related grief that was bothering me again. Thing is, that year, it was my mother.

I was in college, and just trying to get through second semester to get the credits. I had figured out in first semester that Nursing was not the course for me. The only reason I bothered with second was because my mother pressured me. She would have pushed me to continue through the entire thing, seeing as she was already buying the third semester books. I, however, put my foot down. Things were tense between us after that.

That year, I was not dating anyone, but I did screw around with Ian on occasion when the need arose. Honestly, doing that had made me feel awful too. You know what, I'm not meant to be a "friends with benefits" or "no strings attached" kind of woman.

I was in a terrible mood that year. I still thought I had lost a baby two years prior, and then there was the drama with Nick the year before. Add some "dating jealousy" during the most loving time of year, on top of issues with my mother, and I was going downhill, fast. It got to the point that, once the 14th rolled around, I decided to skip class. My mother was working days, so I figured she wouldn't know any better.

I ended up texting a girl in my class that I carpooled with to let her know not to come get me. Ian had messaged me around lunch to wish me a Happy Valentine's Day, and ask why I wasn't in school. I shrugged it off, pretending I was just being a jealous ass that didn't want anything to do with Valentine's Day. It was half-true, back then, after all.

I was in the bath when Mum came home from work in the afternoon. She asked me how my day was, which I answered with a "it was okay". Then she was quiet for a bit.

"Did you go to school today?" she suddenly asked.

"Yeah," I was confused. It seemed like such a random question until I realized my cellphone was downstairs on the kitchen counter.

"Are you sure?" she growled. She also said something more that was basically quoting my excuse to Ian. I can't remember the exact wording, but I was pissed.

Knowing she knew, but still sticking to my guns, I spat, "Yes."

She went silent again. I could hear her storming around the kitchen collecting what she needed to go to her second job. I could tell she was just as angry as I was. Thankfully, she never came into the bathroom. If she did, I'm sure we would have got into an argument. It was one of those days that I would have fought her if she provoked me. Even through a shower curtain.

Finally, as she was leaving, she shouted, "You know, if you're going to lie, you should delete shit off your phone!"

Which is why I do now. It took a couple other invasions of privacy before I finally started to regularly remember to sign out of my facebook, or delete messages, but I got it. Mum had never been one to respect my thoughts or opinions. I thought that at least she had respected my space as far as messages sent to people. I don't know what had compelled her to snoop that day, but that was the first time she had fully crossed the line into fully disrespecting me, and my privacy.

I was 20 going on 21 that year, by the way.

February 14th, 2013... the day that I learned I could not trust my own mother. To this day, I still watch my back. I had forgotten for a little while, but this past August had been a reminder.

I had to take a moment from writing this passage. Clearly, I'm bitter today. It's probably a side effect of all the negativity I've wallowed in for three weeks. I was pretty pissy after my meeting with Dr Adams on Monday. After talking to her about what has happened over the last month and a half, her suggestions were the same as before: diet, exercise, and medication.

It pissed me off that she was pushing pills again. Honestly, I don't want to be on medication. I know my issues are situational, not chemical. I know I am an emotionally sensitive individual. Which means that when I'm happy, I'm a kid with a puppy on Christmas. And when I'm in a negative mood, such as irritable, I am easily set off with everything.

She did make the point, however, that, yes, anti-depressants are not going to solve the problem. It may be what I need to keep away from those extreme lows until I know how to cope without. It was enough to have me consider it. After I had cooled off, of course.

I brought it up with Linda on our Wednesday meeting.

Linda is a stark contrast in how she helps. She reminds me that the negative thoughts I'm having is a learned self-blame. She says I'm putting needless pressure on myself to not fuck up, and that my ideas of failure are also fairly extreme.

A large part of me doesn't want to agree. It says I'm just a lazy ass that is using a serious condition as an excuse to lay around all day. That same voice berates me that I should not be on a reduced course-load. That, if I get my head out of my ass, I would be able to get my certificate with my classmates this year, too.

I talked to Cam too. She says medication will help quiet that horrible inner voice.

Admittedly, there's a small voice that says I should try it. It's not like I can't stop taking the medication if it turns out to be ineffective, or have more negative effects than good.

I am scared to, though. I don't like things that mess with my head. It's why I don't do drugs, or drink, or anything like that. My knowledge, and creativity are really the only things I have going for me. I don't want to loose either of them.

Linda, and Anita, assured me that I would likely be more creative, and be able to concentrate better if I tried medication. Both would be nice. It is tiresome feeling like I'm loosing my mind.

Either way, I have a follow-up appointment with Dr Adams on Wednesday, the 15th. I have until then to think about it. For all I know, something will happen this 14th that will convince me medication might be necessary.

You Are Stronger Than This

Yesterday was Monday the 13th. I started the day in a not so healthy frame of mind. I was avoiding class because I didn't want to face my teacher, but I also did not want to be alone that day. Desperation was telling me to reach out to someone. A friend, my sister, my mother... anybody. It was while I was crying from purely feeling lost and overwhelmed, I decided facing my professor would be easier than battling with my own head all day.

I spent the whole painting class looking at my thrown together diorama. It was honestly just a bunch of things from out of my locker. I couldn't seem to make sense of the instructions I had been given about washing out monochromatic colour. My classmates were hard at work on theirs, but I could not see their works because they were using the painting donkeys with their backs to the wall. I was forced to sit in the middle of the class since there was no more room where my peers were at.

The longer I tried to figure out what the teacher had meant, the more I was doubting my own abilities. Maggie seemed to notice I was getting frustrated as she came over and tried to explain it to me in a different way.

Try as I might, I still could not understand what Maggie meant. She started apologizing that she 'isn't explaining it properly'. This lead me to apologize saying she was explaining fine, I was just not understanding what people were trying to tell me.

By the time lunch had rolled around- which was only a little over an hour since I had arrived late to class- I wanted to go home. My classmates were just being their friendly selves, and I felt like I was intruding with my presence. I had convinced myself that I was not a real artist, and "how dare I, an imposter, try to befriend truly talented people". I had to excuse myself to head for the counselling office in hopes of finding someone to talk through my frustrations and fears.

I was breathless just heading for the stairs let alone climbing them. I had to check my pulse at the top because I was light-headed. My heart rate was super high. Faster than after a long run.

Fat lard. You can't even get up a flight of stairs without giving yourself a heart attack, my more cruel inner voice spat.

I pushed it aside, and hurried on to the counselling room. The office was almost completely empty. Just the pair of receptionists, and a security guard. I was called up to the one, and I asked if there was someone available for triage.

There wasn't.

Not to mention, Linda was off for the day, and Anita was fully booked. I was on my own.

The receptionist was nice enough to provide me with the local crisis calling card. I noticed there was an address on it too. I'll have to see if maybe I should visit it today or tomorrow. I didn't bother with it yesterday, though.

For one thing, despite my hopeless "I'm a giant fuck-up" attitude, I knew it was a phase for the day. I told myself I just needed to calm down. I was not a crisis case. I'm just a girl with poor coping skills.

For another, I did not want to waste time talking to some stranger, explain everything, and then have them push medication at me like Dr Adams is doing. At least the counselling triage at the school has a record of me to work from.

Lastly, I did not want to do anything that would cause me to miss more class. I had the feeling Marla was irritated with me for coming to class with nothing completed. I'm sure my lack of productivity during class time yesterday had pissed her off, too.

Granted, that could just be my self-judgemental side portraying an emotion that may or may not be present in someone else.

Regardless, I did not want to make matters worse by missing any more class time. Even if it was a few minutes just to talk with a counsellor.

Since there was no one to talk to, I went to my fall back: I hid in a bathroom and cried. I was confused why the hell I was being such a cry-baby yesterday. I could not make sense of why I felt like I needed to sob, and whimper like some wounded puppy. Granted, I was able to be a little louder since it was a single toilet bathroom.

It took me about ten minutes before I felt enough relief to look myself in the mirror, and mutter, "you're stronger than this."

I refused to let myself stay there, and whine, any longer than that. I cleaned myself up, and tried to not make any eye contact the entire trek back to the studio. I know it was still obvious I had been crying by the time I got to class. Thankfully, no one said anything about it. Not even just a concerned, "are you okay?", because that was one of those moments any act of kindness might have set me off further. I think they knew that, and that's why we went back to talking like normal.

When class started up again, it was time to do critiques of everyone's works. It's while we were going from painting to painting, giving our feedback, and listening to the teacher explain her own pros and cons to each piece, I suddenly understood what the intrusions had been.

I know now that it's supposed to be a *painterly* piece. A term I had learned the previous semester.

Finally, understanding allowed me to feel more at ease. I even contemplated a different diorama since I have all of reading week to actually make a worth while piece.

Knowing what is expected of me over the next two weeks until our next painting class, and the company of my class friends helped make the day better... ironically, I really did not want to go home when class was finished at 3. People were leaving, though, and I was in need of a nap.

Braving school had worked out for the better. No matter how exhausted I was after the fact. I ended up falling asleep around 5:30 pm- after talking with Cam- and was only woken at 8:30 pm because Nick had called.

He had been texting me since 6, called twice, and even knocked on my door. I had not heard any of it. I'm sure my subconscious had, and that's why I had started waking up enough that I had heard the second phone call. He said he had something for me, but did not say what.

At first I was a little annoyed. I had thought it would be something sexual that would be a 'mutual' gift. Turned out, it was two regular sized packages of lindor chocolate, and a single white rose.

The fucker remembered my favourite flower.

His Valentine's gift was a surprise visit, with some chocolates and flowers. I don't care how damn cliche that is. The reason it is cliche is because it's a sweet gesture. I am all for creativity as much as the next girl, but there is absolutely nothing wrong with the classics.

I think I am more glad for the surprise company. No one takes the time to come visit me without some long term planning before hand. Probably to give me a heads up to make sure my place is properly cleaned for company.

Nick's unexpected company after a rough day was greatly appropriated. The gifts were just the bonus material. Better still, his company was just that. We talked about games, and movies. There was no pressure about sex. Even when we went to bed for the night at midnight.

It wasn't until we woke up at quarter after 4 am that he started to get more touchy-feelly. I didn't want to, though. I was actually get pissed off at his advances.

Did he think I now owe him a favour because he wanted to be romantic for Valentine's Day? I should have stuck with my original instinct when I answered the door. It's always about sex with him. Always.

I politely declined.

He apparently figured that meant intercourse only, and was trying to rub off on me. I was going to let him have his fun because I was of the mind, "whatever. It's not sex."

Except, I wasn't having that either. I kept moving away from him. He thought it was a game, but after I kept doing it, he actually got up, and got ready for work. Only, then he stalled. He said he was debating calling in to "just snuggle" today. He ended up undressing again, and trying more. I was trying to be nice by reminding him that he should be going to work.

"I will. I just want to have a little fun first," was his response.

As he persisted, I moved away, "Okay. You've had you're *little bit* of fun."

He chuckled, "What? Not going to help a guy out?"

"I don't want the mess," I said in the same tone he had just used to ask his question.

He persisted a little more, and finally I told him, "Stop. You've had your fun, but I don't feel like doing this."

He shrugged it off as PMS, but, thankfully, he did not continue. He got dressed again, and headed out for work. I'm sure his "poor blue balls" is going to annoy him today. Good for him.

As for me, I feel quiet empowered this morning. I faced down an anxiety day, and still managed to function as a student. And, I stood against one of Nick's advances.

I think I'll count this as one of the better Feburary 14th memories. Happy Valentine's Day.

Bonding

It's Tuesday, February 21st. I have been at my mother's house since Friday. Right now she's taking the dog to the groomer, so I thought I would do some writing.

I can't say her attitude is any different than normal during my extended stays. I can, however, say this experience has been different.

For one thing, this is my 6th day on my new anti-depression medication. I know I've been fighting it. It was my needless crying on the 13th that finally leaned the scale in favour of giving it a try. It ended up being the perfect timing. If I'm going to test an anti-depressant on how well it can keep me balanced in high stress situations, visiting my mother for nearly a week will do the trick.

I found myself super hyper on Friday. The same giddy, giggly sensation I get when I've downed too much candy, or haven't slept in over 20 hours. On a positive note, Mum and I had spent our time in London laughing up a storm. She had wanted to do a little bit of shopping.

We were going through various thrift and outlet stores just to see what was out there. I had been cracking several jokes, but the one that stuck began in the Goodwill in downtown London. Mum was skimming the clothing racks, and stopped in front of the pyjamas. She pulled out the leg of what honestly had to be the ugliest shade of lilac. I didn't know any shade of purple could look so terrible.

"Don't these look comfy," she grins.

In my opinion, no they did not. They were ruffled and thin. I reached out to touch it when she prompted me to. I thought maybe it was one of those pairs that was deceptively soft. Sure enough, the fabric was rough.

"Feels like a curtain," I shrug. In my mind, the feel, colour, and ruffles were far better suited for some little old lady's bathroom sheers than to be worn as nightwear.

Mum eyed me with her, "are you serious?" look. I countered with my super cheese-y false grin, knowing that would get her to scoff, and smile. Instead, she started to laugh. When it sunk in what I had said, in the tone I had said it, I started giggling too.

"You're such an ass," she tried to scoff like normal, but it came out as a snicker. We were still chuckling all the way out of the store.

Fast forward two or three stores, and we are in this outlet store. It some sort of home decor place with furniture, paintings, and various other household items. There was even a spot with giant throw rugs hung on display in the same manner as one would pick out a poster. I, of course, was instantly drawn to the brightest rug in the bunch. I knew Mum thinks my taste in vibrant colours, especially when home decor is concerned, is obnoxious.

Of course I shout out, "Hey, Mum, look!"

She sets her eyes on my find, and shakes her head. I know she said something because I saw her mouth move, but I was not close enough to hear. She then wanders off to another isle. I thought she had gone into the one next to it, since it had pillows and bedding, and we were apparently on the hunt for stuff for my sister's apartment. Turns out, she had gone into the isle that was entirely curtains.

I could not help myself. I squeezed between the clothing rack so that I could come out beside her. I reached out to touch the curtain she was feeling; which was actually softer than the freaking pyjama pants. Then, with a mischievous grin on my face I look up at her.

She beat me to the punch-line, though. "Feels like pyjamas."

She even used the same, completely serious tone I had used prior. We burst out in fits of laughter.

And THEN, we reached our final store. This one was all clothing. By the time we reached that store, my hyper spell was starting to wind down. I was getting sleepy, and ready to relax for the coming hour and a half long ride to Chatham.

As the two of us wandered up and down the displays, my eyes fell on a white blouse. It was the exact same thin, ruffled material that the pants had been made of. I call for Mum's attention, and pull a sleeve from the rack. As soon as she sees it, she looks me dead in the eye.

"Feels like a curtain." I'm not sure how I was able to stay straight faced, and serious to deliver the line, but I did. And it was hilarious.

The joke had reached full circle when Mum said her famous line again, "You're such an ass."

She says that a lot to my sister and I when either of us make jokes that catches her off guard. That's kind of how the relationship between the three of us works. When all of us are in a good mood, we start to badger one another.

For example, Mum had watched this video online about a little boy who had taken a cupcake. The boy's mother is clearly the one recording, and she's at him about taking the cupcake just to get him flustered. I don't blame the mother because this three or four year old suddenly starts going, "Listen. Listen, Linda. Linda, you're not listening to me."

Because of this video, any time Cam and I would pester her in a way she did not find funny, she would growl, "Listen, Linda." It was her way of making clear she's annoyed, but trying not to ruin our fun since she does the same right back at us.

After a while, she did not even have to include "Linda" for us to know what she was making reference to. This left an opening for us to turn her reference back on her.

"Listen," Mum snipped.

"Linda," I supplied. Cam and I started to giggle more.

Mum does not usually have a comeback to that one.

I get as good as I give, though. A couple years back I had been nice enough to make the three of us lunch. It was just cooked noodle coated in butter, but that was a norm for us when wanting to make a quick, easy lunch. The thing is, when I made it, I had used a fork instead of a knife to separate a chunk of butter from the stick. The result was that the next time Mum went to us it, she was stunned.

"What did you do, bite it?" I explained that I used a fork, but Mum continued, "It looks like perfect teeth marks." She then imitated a beaver gnawing on a log.

That's when the joke about "Bucky the butter biter" started. I can take the jokes about 'butter biting' because it's completely ridiculous. Which is why Cam has learned to only make reference to that side of it. Like the time she came to London with groceries Mum had bought for me. In the mix was a stick of butter.

"Try not to bite it," she teased.

"Well there goes my dinner plan," I laughed back.

I'm not a fan of the 'Bucky' part though. They just added it to make an alliteration, but it bothers me. While growing up, my adult teeth had a habit of coming in long before my baby teeth would fall out. The result was that, at one time, I had four front teeth.

It was at that self conscious age. I'm sure that, had I been a little older, my extra teeth would have been just another thing I would have been bullied about.

They had eventually fallen out, and I do, thankfully, have a straight set of teeth without ever needing braces.

Thus, being called "Bucky" would bring back that self-aware concern.

Oh, and something else different about this visit. Since my sister has officially moved into her new place, I was able to sleep over there twice. The first sleep over was planned. We hung out Saturday night, though I did not learn until the same day that she had also invited Tony, Kev, and Joe.

So much for our sister time, I had thought.

It turned out to be good though. We played some *Mario Kart*, and then, while the others played *Super Smash Brothers*, I turned on my *Pokemon Go* app. It turned out one of my favourites was in the vicinity. The moment I said out loud that it was in the area, Kev got excited too. Suddenly, the two of us were heading off a good 5 or 6 blocks to a church I didn't even know was there. It's a wonder the radar even picked up the stop from the distance we had to cover.

It was quite enjoyable to be out "on an adventure", as Kev called it. It had been a long time since he and I had hung out just the two of us. We chat, and laughed, and compared the latest facts we had learned about this or that. Hilariously, we were speed walking not only to get there before the Pokemon disappeared, but also before BOTH of our phones died.

We made it in time. Then, not even 5 paces down the street returning to my sister's apartment, both phones instantly died. It could not have been more perfectly timed. Something we both had a hoot about.

Honestly, I hope I can hang out more with Kev again. He is my best friend since elementary school. We have grown to be very different people, but we always had different opinions to begin with. That was the beauty of our friendship while we were growing up. Having him as my friend forced me to think outside of my optimistic dreamer mindset.

The Runaway

Predictably, I was pulled away from my writing by my mother. We ended up having a BBQ for dinner tonight. Probably because I had suggested it two days ago as something easier to make than the meal Mum had planned that day. She was in a bit of a mood, which is why I was trying to make things simpler.

My mind had wandered while I was BBQing, and settled on a memory from long ago. It had happened in the dead of winter. Mum had said we would watch a movie together when she got home from work. The house was not clean enough for her, however, upon coming home. She spent a good twenty to thirty minutes screaming her usual speech about how she works so much, and why can't we get off our lazy asses and actually help out around the house.

Somewhere in that rant she had said something along the lines of, "why should I waste my time watching a movie with you guys when I have other shit to do."

She then proceeded to demand we do her bidding for the next hour. After which, we could watch the movie. Truth be told, I would have preferred to hide in my room after to stay away from her.

The more she breathed down our necks, the angrier I got. My sister and I would share looks showing our solidarity. Low grumbles about why Mum couldn't open her eyes, and see all that we had done that day.

After our hour sentence was up, we all gathered downstairs. Mum had to make herself a tea before coming down first, though. When she finally came down, she snipped, "Why haven't you put the movie in yet?"

I don't know what drove me to do it, but I snapped back, "Are you sure we wouldn't be wasting your time?"

I don't remember what was said after that. I just remember

Mum shouting at me. I remember running upstairs to shove my school uniform into my book bag, and then running out the door. I didn't have my winter jacket, though.

Most of all, I remember the frightened look in my sister's eyes. She would have been too young to remember the fights with Richard. Maybe she remembered the ones with Nicholas since this blow up happened only a couple years after Mum left him. Either way, that look still haunts me.

That night I had initially gone to hide at my elementary school. I have no idea why I had picked there. I suppose I must have thought I had no where to go, and so the treeline along the side fence was the best option to stay. At least it would provide some cover from the snow.

I was there for a long time. Long enough for my hot anger to ebb away, and for me to feel the winter cold seeping through my sweater. At one time, I had seen car lights pull into the school parking lot, but I had chosen to stay hidden. I have no idea if that was Mum, or if someone else may have spotted me, and was just checking what they had seen.

A while after it drove away, I decided I needed a warmer and more secure place to stay. I turned to Kev. He lived with his grandmother in a house even closer to the school than my mother's. I must have been a sight when I showed up on his doorstep. I don't remember the conversation, but I know I was blubbering up a storm.

I was not there long when there was a knock on the door. It turned out to be my mother, who got the address from my sister. I can remember cowering low behind the chair arm in hopes she would not see me through the window. I know I was begging whoever was going to answer the door to not give me up. I think it was Kev's grandmother, though, so she did the adult thing and let my mother in.

I know I tried to beg Kev with my eyes to convince his grandmother to not make me go. Trouble was, he had no more power than I did at that age.

Mum tried to tell me the reason she had come looking for me was because she realized I didn't have my winter jacket. Since she was already spending the time looking for me to give it to me, she decided to just take me home to 'talk'.

Basically, I got a one sided rant again about what a little shit I am, and then grounded.

I think the memory was triggered from something she had said the other day. I was looking at her new calendar. This month is of a young family next to a small snowman they had built.

"Hey, Mum. Do you remember the time Cam and I made a giant snowman when we lived at Nicholas'? The bottom ball was so big you had to come out to help us push it."

"No. I don't remember that kind of shit," she deadpanned. "You guys had a horrible childhood, remember?"

"Says who?" I scoff.

"Both of you. You said it all the time when you were younger."

I think it was that line that caused me to think so much that I felt I needed to write today, instead of waiting until I was home tomorrow. I wanted to come back with, "all teenagers think their lives suck", but... well...

I don't think I would consider my mother or the environment she provided us as abusive. She has done, and continues to do, so much for my sister and I. She truly loves us. Which makes it hard to have a healthy relationship with her.

Do I trust she isn't going to turn around, and say something belittling? How can I be open with her about my life when I know she'll negatively judge me?

It's like I'm still that little girl, hiding in the snow. Do the headlights on me signal anger, or kindness? Even after all these years, I really don't know.

An Idea

24th of February. I'm just waking up, and it's almost noon. I'm still kind of tired. I think this medication is making me even more lethargic than I already, naturally, am.

That's not why I'm writing this passage today for.

Wednesday afternoon. I was quite happy, and confident in myself that day. In my positive state of mind the other day, I decided I was going to invite Nick over for sushi and hang out. I was not going to give into him, and I was going to make sure he left the same night.

Dinner went great. We came back to my place and binge watched some TV shows. The thing is, he fell asleep on the couch by midnight. I decided against waking him. I also chose to stay up as long as I could to avoid his usual play of waiting until we go to bed to start making moves.

I ended up going to bed after 2:30 AM. He, of course, followed. That late at night, however, I was asleep within minutes. Well worth offsetting my sleeping pattern to be too tired for his games.

I was jolted awake by his alarm. He got a little too hands on for my liking. I countered by pulling away, and wrapped the covers around me. He lingered in the bed far too long. I was starting to wonder if he was going to pull his, "I can be late for work" routine.

He didn't, though.

"Did you just call in?" I sleepily ask him.

He cuddles up close, "Yeah. I just wanted to spend the day with you."

My blood instantly boils. I get up, grab two of the blankets, and two of my pillows, and move to the couch. I tell him I'm too hot, and need to cool off with the open patio door. Lucky it's nice weather outside.

The nerve. He did not ask me if I was up for company. He was already over-staying his welcome by being there through the night. It took me some time to cool off, but I was, thankfully, still tired. Enough so that I slept until 11-11:30 AM. I was woken up by my mother texting me.

Nick ended up leaving me be until after I had got up to use the bathroom. I went back to laying on the couch because there is not enough room for two people to lay side by side on it. We ended up chatting for a bit, and then I decided I wanted my bed. Between sleeping on my sister's couch for two nights, the rock hard twin bed at my mother's, and then sharing my bed until I went to sleep on my own couch, I just wanted the space to comfortably sprawl out.

It was while I was heading back to bed that I decided I was going to tell Nick to leave when I had to go to my appointment at 2 pm. I ended up relaxing like I wanted, while he was trying to be tender by giving me a message. I was not going to turn that down.

1:30 rolled around, and I got up to get ready without any incident with him. I knew there was a side of me that wanted to give in. Which made me worry my idea yesterday was going to back fire on me. But I held my ground against both him and myself.

All doubts in myself left during my meeting with Linda. She told me I was proving that I was making progress in the way I was talking about this visit to Chatham. How I didn't react to Mum's anger over the missed phone call as a personnel attack. I did not react in my usual way... anxious to please her, or angry and ready to fight. I felt the fear, and then the anger trying to bury it, but I did not react with either way.

Linda reminded me of how I was when she first met me.

"At the time, you were hopeless, and did not think you had it in you to do anything."

As soon as she said it, I remembered the details of the day I first met her. At the time, I was sure I would fail my classes.

I was sure that my family only tolerated me. I was sure that I am too broken of a person for friends and love. I didn't believe in myself.

Has it really only been 4-5 months that I've started to believe in life again?

I know I still get frustrated with myself, and overwhelmed with normal life stresses. Right now, though, I'm only slightly behind in my classes. I have actually attended more classes in these last couple of weeks than I had all of last semester. Which also means I'm more comfortable with my classmates.

Right now, things are good with my sister and I. There is a part of me waiting for her to turn on me when her birthday comes around, but at the same time, she is another year older. Maybe she's gained some new insights in the last year. Maybe our relationship is better right now, enough that we will continue to get along more and more.

Things are still rocky with my mother, but I'm reacting differently. I'm understanding more, and we're working things out. I think the distance between us helps because now I can live, and learn by making my own choices.

I have been growing more and more into myself. Who am I, and what I want to do with my life. I know I'm still going to stress, and have my days where I feel like I cannot do things. But I know now that it's not just me over-reacting. I suffer from mental health, and that doesn't make me weak or stupid or a failure. It just means I've gone through some shit, and it's taken it's tole on my mind. It's made me insecure, distrusting, and hopeless. But that's okay. It doesn't have to define me. It's just something I have to live with, no different than someone living with an amputated limb.

I'm still breathing.

Living Nightmares

Today is March 13th. I seem to have hit a mental wall that has resulted in a relapse in my depression. The result is that I have no interest in doing anything. It's lucky I get up and actually eat something in a day, let alone go to school, exercise, or clean.

I have had plenty of opportunities to even just journal. Every time I tried, I would end up staring at the screen, and crying. The cruelest inner voices ripping me down at every waking moment. It's to the point that, once again, I have no will to be awake.

It does not help any that I had to stop taking my medication. I can say there was definitely a difference being on it and not. The issues arose after I started taking the full doses. The longer I was on it, the more lethargic and nauseated I became. By the Friday before last, I was starting to vomit. I thought it was just a bug, at first, and so continued, but two days later, I stopped the medication.

I was terrified that the combination of not being able to remain awake, and continuous emptying of what little was in my stomach would become life threatening. People can suffocate in their sleep from vomiting, and not being aware enough to turn over.

My mind would have preferred to chance death. At least I would have fallen asleep, and not been any wiser that I have passed until I stand before Heaven's gate. This suffering would have been over.

Instead, I'm at war within myself once more.

I started thinking that I have no work ethic. *You're a dreamer only, and will never amount to anything. It's just dead-end after dead-end, no matter what I do. Nothing you do will ever be enough. You just get tired, and give up.*

It came down to, "Why am I trying then?"

That's about the point the second part started to kick in. I stopped dreaming. I stopped hoping. I just went completely numb because thinking about things that made me happy was torture. The alternative is to let myself feel every ache inside, and wish for death.

That is probably the major point that kept me away from writing. As I write about what I'm feeling, I think about how people would react.

"Oh, she's just an emo. She just needs to learn to be thankful for what she has. There are people in the world with a lot less."

There is a twinge of anger because I know that has nothing to do with anything. If anyone bothered to get to know me, they would know how hard I am trying. I'm not an angry soul with a chip on my shoulder. I'm just someone that's been through shit, and I'm tired. I have no more hope to get me out of bed.

You want to know what depression is really like?

It's loneliness when you're in a room full of loved ones. You convince yourself that they don't actually care about you. You feel like you're an obligation that should just learn to stop trying to push your presence on others. Eventually, you swing back and forth between quietly avoiding others so as not to burden them, or doing everything in your power to make people know how much you appreciate them.

At the same time, I feel like I'm being an attention whore, or I'm too clingy. Even when I'm by myself, and want to talk to someone, I don't because I don't want to push them away from being overly emotional.

It's believing you don't deserve to be happy. You haven't done enough to earn your dreams, and you're suffering is punishment for ever thinking otherwise.

It's telling yourself that you are a failure at everything. You could be talented enough of a painter to fully recreate the

Sistine Chapel on a quarter. But you would still think that you're a shit painter, and "how unoriginal that you had to copy a real artist's work". I know I can write, but then the whisper starts.

Any loser can put words on a piece of paper and call it a story. That doesn't mean what I've written is actually something worth reading.

It's a need to constantly keep your brain busy, because if you don't, you'll be haunted by every moment of fear, embarrassment, guilt, and anger you have ever experienced in your life. An uncontrollable inferno trapping you in random, chaotic thoughts. You feel these memories like it's happening all over again. Avoiding it is impossible, because there will always be the quiet moments. Like when you're in the shower, or when you're trying to fall asleep. Suddenly, boredom is a poison towards a long and slow death to your soul.

The perfect example was the last couple of nights. Each time I closed my eyes, I was a little kid again.

At first, it was Heart and Stroke awareness week, and we were given skipping ropes to do work outs. The other kids could not say anything in phys. ed. class, but during recess, it was just so hilarious to watch the 'fat lard' try to jump rope. I remember being told once that I could not join the other girls in my class for a round of jump rope because I might step on the rope, and end up breaking it.

You see, that little bit just triggered another memory. It's a cool morning at school. The majority of my classmates are lined up to take turns trying to shoot a hoop. I'm walking with my shoulders slouched, keeping close to the brick wall. I want to join them, but I know they would never allow it. I'm stuck longingly watching.

If that wasn't bad enough, I suddenly notice many of them are watching me. They are whispering to one another. I try to feign courage by straightening my back, and meeting their stares. Then, all of a sudden, the girls start to shriek and there is a chorus of "ew"s.

"Why don't you watch where you are walking?!" one girl shouts.

It was only then I realized I had stepped on a used condom. Honestly, who leaves something like that in an elementary school yard?

I wish I could say things were better at home, but they weren't. The other night, as I had to get up to use the bathroom, I remembered a ridiculous rule when living at Nicholas'. The rule was that we could not get out of bed for anything without asking permission first. That included using the toilet.

It was only directed at us girls because Cody needed the exception.

I can remember crawling out of bed one night, and calling out for Nicholas. Mum was at work, and I could hear the TV playing in the living room. I dare not leave the threshold of the little bedroom. He was not above smacking us for rule breaking. Despite desperately calling out to him for 20 or 30 minutes, he never answered. I ended up wetting my pajamas. I can still clearly remember they were purple with little lambs on them.

I knew I could not go back to bed in piss covered clothing. Mustering what courage I could, I finally ventured out. It turns out, he had been asleep on the couch. I can still hear his voice booming the moment he opens an eye, and sees that I'm out of bed. It only get's worse when I try to explain what happened. I ended up spanked, and told I was an idiot for not just running to the bathroom. He kept calling me a baby, and 'asked' if he was going to need to put me in diapers.

I remember trying to not cry too loudly as I hide beneath my covers after Mum came home, and Nicholas was telling her what I had done.

There was another time that I was trying to not cry too

loud. Mum and Nicholas were fighting over something. I was trying to keep Cam distracted because I knew if either of us made a peep, Nicholas' ire would increase. I was terrified he would hit my mother because of me. I convinced Cam we should drape a blanket from the top bunk to turn the bottom one into a fort.

We sat in the corner of that dark little fort. I can still feel my sister against my side. There's a book in my hand, but it's closed because I'm trying to shush her.

Nightmare after nightmare, I can't get away from any of it. I just wish it would stop. How do I make it stop?

Invasion of Privacy

I found out this past Friday that my mother has, apparently, been tracking my text messages. Even though I pay the bill, it's under her name. Back when I got the phone I knew it would be a bad idea. At that time, I asked to have the billing under my own name.

Mum, however, had a contract through her job that meant I got my phone and bill at a discount price. At the time, I figured the only control this would give Mum is for her to suddenly cancel it on me. What had never occurred to me was that she could call the phone provider to see what numbers I call or text, and when.

I don't know the full extent of the information she can get her hands on. At best, that means she knows I text Nick. Which, oh well, she already knew since August. She still can't face me about it because then she would have to admit she's invaded my privacy to learn I'm talking to him.

At worst, she can read every text message I have ever sent. Every time I've vented to someone about crap; especially the crap she puts me through. Everything someone has ever told me. I mean, the worst she's going to get from my comments to Nick is dirty texts, or arrangements to meet up.

It just fucking pisses me off. I had to call my Aunt Heather to know if Mum had said anything to her that indicated how long she has been doing this, and how much she knows.

She's doing it to Cam as well. Mum had bitched to Grandma about how often I'm in contact with Nick, and mentioned she could see Cam's too. Despite Mum telling them not to say anything, both my grandparents agreed what Mum is doing is invasive, and bullshit. They told my sister. Thus, Cam called Friday to tell me.

It wouldn't look weird for her to call because she and I

have been calling each other a lot for the last couple of weeks. My relationship with her is actually really good right now.

The thing is, neither Cam nor I can call Mum out on invading our privacy because it will come back on Grandma.

Utter bullshit.

If I had not spoken to Aunt Heather, I probably would have broke by now, and blew up at my mother. It's just one more thing she's done to me. One more way she's trying to control my life. During my initial rage over the situation, I came to question if I want to have a relationship with my mother.

As it sits, I'm only allowed to have her in my life if I play by her rules. Those rules include not being allowed to talk about my writing, or other interests.

It made me realize just how much I suppress of myself. I stopped going to church because she hated me going. She still refers to Christians as "wack-jobs", "nut cases", or "bible thumpers". She treated my decision to follow God like me saying I joined some cult or drug gang.

To be honest, I think she would have preferred if I was some drug gang member.

I have nicknames like "the walking encyclopedia of useless knowledge" because I like learning about how the world works. Since these are things she doesn't care about, it's all 'useless' knowledge, and I need to stop talking about it.

She kept taking me to concerts because I'm supposed to like them because she likes them. No matter how many times I made clear to her that they make me miserable.

Just like none of the ideas I had for a future career were good enough. Anything I said was ripped apart to show me I'm just being a stupid dreamer. Until, finally, I picked the job she wanted; Registered Practical Nursing. I couldn't even pick what college I wanted to attend. No, it had to be the same college she had gone to.

You know, I had to really fight with her to be allowed to go to Ursuline College Secondary School instead of George McGregor High School. McGregor was, of course, her high school. Just like how St Ursula was her elementary school. Didn't matter there were way better elementary schools in the area that would have actually challenged me academically. I had to attend the same one she did, no matter how much it became underfunded.

I get it. She had me when she was 19. Her whole world/self-purpose was shaped around raising my sister and I. Giving us all the things she never had. All except the one thing that counted most of all; our freewill.

She hated our father so much that any traits that came out similar to him, or his side of the family, had to go. She had baptized me Catholic, so I was to either practice Catholicism, or nothing at all. Especially not Christianity (yes, there's a difference).

Making silly voices and accents? I still can't do them around her.

That's just a couple of examples. I'm tired of questioning myself just for my mother's approval. I know the reason I constantly second guess myself is because I was never allowed to think for myself. Any time I ever had an idea, she would tell me why it was wrong.

I couldn't tell her I was starting to get depressed back in grade 10. It was just winter blues, according to her.

I wasn't allowed to sleep when I wanted to. Because I was (insert age) which means I should be staying up until such and such a time, and still be expected to get up like normal the next morning.

I'm tired of her being controlling. I'm sick of second guessing myself because I don't know what's me, and what is just trying to please my mother.

I know she's my Mum, but I don't want her in my home. I

don't want her in my life. As incredibly sad as that is to say, I've let her hold power over me for so long.

I'm done reaching out to her first just so we actually have a conversation. I'm done with being interrupted, or not being allowed to have an opinion. I'm sick of being stabbed in the back, and feeling like I have to bend to her will just to have her in my life.

I'm tired of being told I'm so ungrateful, and treated like I'm the worst just because I don't bend to her every beck and call.

I could just be super pissed off right now. Plus, it doesn't help that the first time I hear from her since reading week was to bitch about a costume she will never wear.

Mum, "Hey was going through closet downstairs and wondering if next time you come home if you can dig out the gown part of my nun costume please. Would like to put all away together."

Mum, "How's it going up there? How is school? Any luck finding a job? Did you get computer?"

Annie, "99.99% sure I already gave it back when I gave you the puzzle. Will check for it anyway."

Annie, "Not great. Going through a really bad depression episode, but working through. Trust me, if I get a job, you will likely be the first person I text to celebrate."

Mum, "Nope you said you had to find it."

That was it. I couldn't even respond because that fucking costume means so much more to her than me. I really wanted to come back with, "well, if I go through with killing myself, you'll be able to go through my things as proof that I don't have it."

Great, I'm now emotionally exhausted, and I still have to go to get cat food. I suppose I could use the distraction.

Choices

It's 3 am on March 19th. With another week behind me, I've had a little more time to recuperate from the low I was at. I still feel like the bottom of an outhouse, but I'm slowly making my way out of this mental shit pile.

Among the many things that happened this week, one thing included was another appointment with Linda. I had seen her the Thursday before, but nothing said had got through. I seemed to be in this spiral because I did not feel like fighting anymore.

I'm sure that, if I were facing this alone, I would have gone with curling up, and let myself slip away.

But I'm not alone.

Linda was asking me to consider withdrawing from the semester. Tomorrow (the 20th) is the last day to decided without any draw backs.

The mere thought sent me into a panic. I don't know if I can finish the semester with an above 65% average. If I don't, I won't be able to return come September.

Yet, the alternative feels far worse to me. It means I would have to see a new counsellor. I really don't want to have to revisit things I am trying to put behind me so that some new person would understand. It means loosing contact with the handful of people I have been gaining a friendship with.

Let's face it, I'm terrible about staying in touch unless I see someone regularly. It's just this mindset of, "I don't want to bother so-and-so," and then morphs into a, "They probably don't even consider me a friend, anyway."

Of course, withdrawing leaves me with an uncertain future. I have no doubt OSAP will want the remaining money returned to them. I need that to survive at least another month until I either get a job, or I can apply for OW again.

Trust me when I say, I *really* want to avoid Ontario

Works, again.

You know, I started this passage with the intent to consider if I should withdraw from school or not. I mean, on Thursday I was so determined to not let that happen that I secretly went to talk to my Professor after my meeting with Linda. Just to explain that, yes I'm having a hell of a time, but I desperately want to try.

Not sure if that was me being brave, or me just trying to survive.

I have 2 1/2 projects that I'm supposed to be working on to have completed for tomorrow. That didn't seem like much until I'm actually facing it down. I may have the pastel piece completed, but I can't guarantee the paintings.

I have no one to blame for my desperate situation than myself. Which is why I need to fix it, myself, too.

I think there are some pretty obvious answers to a handful of choices that I have before me.

The Dragon Egg

    I did make it to my painting class yesterday. I was late, and I had to excuse myself for an hour long appointment with Dr Adams. Still, I went. I spent the whole day in the same subdued low that I've been through over the last couple of weeks. I spent the entire time longing for home. Not even socializing seemed to help.

    It doesn't help any that I've been restless. It's like I want to run off somewhere. Just put a pause on life and escape from all worries. Thank goodness camping season is opening up soon.

    I don't believe this is wander lust, though. It's more a need to recollect myself without worrying about bills and school work.

    I'm left rather sleepless. It's a record low for me to get only 3-5 hours of sleep a night. Further more, my body has resorted to painful reminding me to actually eat each day. I have a few items in my cupboards. I just have no interest in cooking, eating, or clean-up afterwards. It's already nearly noon, and I've only just had what will likely be the only meal of my day.

    So why starve myself? I don't know, ask my depression. It's fucking stupid in my opinion.

    My meeting with Dr Adams was interesting, to put it lightly. She was trying to prompt me to talk since I wasn't saying much. I just updated her on the crap with my mother.

    Dr Adams switched gears, and asked me to name what I want to do. If my mental health was in the right place, where would I see myself in the future?

    It would appear that question pushed the water works button. I swear, I've been crying way to much lately.

    The most frustrating part is that, when I'm so overwhelmed, crying, and need to get out what's on my mind, is when I find myself incapable of speech. It's like I can't think words, but I'm still thinking at the speed of light.

On a good note, it's started a running joke between Linda and I. When one of us can't seem to find the right thing to say, we say, "words are hard."

Dr Adams does not know this joke, so I can't cut the tension I'm feeling by spouting it out. Thankfully, she had thought to hand me a pen and paper when it got too bad to speak. I don't know what magic is involved that decides I can still formulate words and sentence structure to write in times that talking is impossible, but I am grateful.

I left with a new prescription in hand. Hopefully this one will be kinder to my stomach.

My energy was zapped. I had set up my painting supplies before leaving for the appointment, but upon returning, I was unable to paint. That was not fun, by the way. I mean, I actually show up for class, and do nothing. I may have been waving around a flag and shouting, "look at me! I'm a giant fuck up!"

Sure, I don't think anyone actually cared. Linda tells me I have to let it go when I start to think I'm secretly being negatively judged. I'm not a mind reader, after all.

I went home, and slept. I ended up missing my appointment with Anita yesterday, come to think of it. We were supposed to meet for 6 pm. Instead, I was laying in bed, trying to stay alert enough to respond to Nick's text messages to get across the point that I did not want company. There was a couple of times where I had accidentally hit a button, and then would wake up and have to erase the typos.

The last thing I wrote was, "going to have a snooze".

Except what I texted was, "I'm going to snoorlgl." Yeah, I don't know how I ended up with that either.

I did end up sleeping for a solid 4 hours. It was a deep sleep too, because my throat was sore in a way that meant I had to have been snoring. Or talking. I've been told that I tend to talk in my sleep if I'm exceptionally stressed.

All that aside, since I couldn't sleep, and was emotionally drained, I figured I should have a read through my earlier passage. I ended up reading the ones that were meant to be a message to future- now current- me. The whole, "don't give up. You are loved. Whatever you're going through is temporary."

It actually did just as I had hoped it would when I wrote it. It touched the part of me that remembers being hopeful, and happy about what tomorrow brings. It was like having past me tap my shoulder.

"Excuse me," she said. "Just want you to know that you've got this."

My inner critic briefly piped in. Not to smash this bit of lightness I've been reminded can exist inside me. Instead, she was apparently thinking I needed a better metaphor than glass panels, or coal into diamonds.

Yellow butterflies are supposed to represent Mental Health Awareness, she quipped.

"I am NOT resorting to a butterfly in a chrysalis cliche," I outwardly grumbled. All the while I was also trying to focus on drawing a ghost dragon for class. "Besides, they would be destroyed in a fire."

It doesn't have to be a literal butterfly. Are you a fantasy writer, or not?

"Adventure-Fantasy," I corrected. "Butterflies don't make great protagonists or even familiars in those." But then I paused as I looked down at my reference photo once again. "But a dragon is."

I started thinking about how most stories say that dragon eggs hatch from extreme heat. It's possible that I'm inside a dragon's egg. Then the blaze isn't trying to destroy me, or shape me into something new. It's just there to prepare me for whatever lies ahead.

Facing this inferno doesn't feel so terrible when I started thinking about it like that. I'm under pressure and at the mercy of my mental fire because I haven't 'hatched' yet. This is only the beginning of my adventures.

Not to mention, dragon scales are impervious to fire. It's comforting to think that, even though it will be there, I won't be effected by it anymore.

For now, I'm still breathing. Even if it brings me to tears to think about right now, I can still dream. Most importantly, there will be a tomorrow.

Making a Come Back

It's 5 am on the 23rd. I'm actually rather hopeful for today.

Firstly, I have an interview with an employment agency. They help those with mental health, and other disabilities, find work. Linda had suggested this place to me because she used to work there. I think having a job that understands I will have low days will be great. It's something to do, I can interact with people, and, of course, have an income to ensure I can make ends meet. Fingers crossed that all goes well.

Secondly, I did cave and buy groceries, yesterday. A bill of almost $200 is the most expensive trip I have ever done, but now I'm good for another two months. Which is why I'll be cooking up a full meal later tonight. It's long over due between lack of supplies, and lack of motivation.

I also stocked up on plenty of easy to make items for those days I don't have the energy to cook. Yesterday was one of them. At least I had cheese and crackers to munch on.

A full stomach isn't the only thing improving my mood. It appears the new medication is working great. I'm not nauseated at all like the first one. We'll see how things go once I'm up to the full dosage, but fingers crossed.

Last thing for today. I have another project finished, and ready to be handed in today. I made serious progress on another, AND I even did some writing last night.

I am feeling really good right now. I'm sure I'll be exhausted by the time the day is done, but I felt I need to write a mini-celebration for future me to read.

See Annie? You're making great progress. I believe in you!

Paper Cranes

March 28th. I'm trying to make small adjustments in my life to help make things better. One of them is to consistently get up at 7 am. Should I wake before that, I force myself to stay quiet in bed, and just listen to outside.

There is a lot going on outside now too. It seems Mother Nature has finally decided on a season this week, and that season is Spring. We are actually starting to get highs among double digits. I think yesterday was 12oC, but I'm not entirely sure.

Perhaps it's the nice weather. Perhaps it's the combination of my new medication and actually putting needed vitamins into my body, but right now I feel calm. More accurately, I'm not dipping down into a horrible state of mind again. The depression side doesn't feel like it's there as much.

I wish I could say the same for the anxiety.

Don't get me wrong. I did spend Friday through Sunday morning mostly sleeping. I think it was just a need to rest. That's what I told myself when the little voice told me I was being lazy.

I ended up making a little rhyme to counter it:

Through troubles and days, you do only your best.
But, when comes the times, you are allowed to rest.

I am attempting other changes too. I'm trying to get myself to clean daily. Right now, I'm pacing myself at only ten minutes each morning. It's a steadily work in progress. This morning it was taking out my trash. I plan to take out the recyclables too since I still have energy.

I'm probably producing more energy too since I made the decision to start using the stairs at random.

Let's be clear, by the way. I am almost 270 lbs of woman, and I live in a high rise. It's not just one or two flights of stairs.

Despite the quaking in my knees, and being winded, I'm quite pleased with myself every time I make it to my floor. I know making that climb a little bit each day is good for me. Eventually, I'll be able to do it without feeling so winded.

I bought a new litter box the other day, too. This one sifts the litter instead of me scooping. It's going to save me some time and effort. I think the only thing better would be a self cleaning one. Though I don't know how the girls would handle one of those self-scooping shit-er boxes.

On the note of making my home more presentable, Mum might be coming to visit me this weekend. I know I'm going to get 20 (cough-thousand-cough) questions, but I'm trying to remind myself that she's just concerned. Yes, she's controlling, but that's because that's her coping mechanism. I know she hates it that I'm suffering inside my own head. She just wants to save me from it. The problem is that she's keeps going about it all wrong.

I'm actually really starting to consider that my Mum has her own anxiety issues as well. Separation anxiety, at the very least.

Okay, now that I've come full circle, there is the issue of my own anxiety.

I have to get some paperwork done to prove to the employment place that I do, in fact, suffer from a mental health disability. Which means I have been waiting since Thursday for Wednesday to have Dr Adams file the paperwork. I was also told that I would hear back from someone once I brought the paperwork in to make an appointment with a case worker.

Basically, all this adds up to is time. The longer I go without a job, the more anxious I am about being able to make my May rent. Which adds onto the fear of being homeless, or having to go back to Chatham. Which adds more pressure on me to finish this semester with a pass so that I can continue with school again in September.

All of this was making me beyond antsy. During my days of rest, however, I realized that Linda was right. I should have withdrawn from this semester, focused on overcoming my mental health, and then have a fresh start at school in the fall. I think I was just scared that I was going to be left alone, without options, and trying to overcome this by myself, again.

That changed yesterday.

On a whim (or a divine intervention, if you will), I decided to go to the Crisis walk-in clinic. I didn't feel like I was in a crisis, but I had just missed another Painting class. This project I won't be able to make up because it involved a live model in class.

I felt lost, and frightened. I knew what I was feeling was the weight of living without existing. It's like, I know I'm alive, and I have to figure out how to keep living, but I have no sense of purpose.

The fact that I feel this way, and I am STILL doing my best leaves me mind boggled. I have no idea where this strength in me to keep going, and to try again, is coming from. I like to think it is God's grace whispering small encouragements inside my soul. Whatever you want to believe it is, I'm grateful it's there.

It was enough to get me out of bed yesterday, put on some clothes, and walk out into the evening air. It was two different bus rides to get to, so I had a lot of time to panic. I wanted to throw up as the second bus drew closer to the destination. Against it all, I still got on those buses, and I still pulled the string to get off at the correct spot instead of just riding it back home.

I was shaking as I put one foot in front of the other to cross that damn parking lot.

What are you doing? That fiery voice started again. *You*

don't actually need help. You're just being weak. You need to get your head out of my ass because Linda and Dr Adams have already told you all the changes you need to make to better your life. What if they decide to institutionalize you because they think you're a risk to yourself? You do realize You're going to have to explain everything all over again. This is going to take forever and it's not going to make a difference.

The moment the receptionist asked how she could help me, my words were caught in my throat.

Run home, idiot! my mind screamed.

Somehow, I mumbled out, "I'm not sure... I-I'm here on a whim..."

The receptionist, Alex, gave me a kind smile, "That's okay. We're glad you came in. Would you like some water?"

I think I smiled while I nodded, but only because I found the offer hilarious. I wonder how many other people ask for water when they go into a mental fit.

We do some talking. I admit that I'm not in crisis, and that I do have appointments on Wednesday and Thursday with established supports.

"Okay, so you're just looking for someone to talk to to get through today," Alex summarized.

I was incredibly surprised because that did make sense. "I think so."

I had to do some paperwork, and while I was, another woman comes in crying. She looked to me like someone that needed this place. They had multiple counsellors, though, so I wasn't worried about if they rushed her in ahead of me like at a hospital.

Apparently, that's not what they do. All walk-ins are considered important so it's in order of who comes in first. Seems like an odd system to me. Though, I understand how another person might feel worse if someone else is put ahead of them.

We were also given the option if we would prefer a male or female counsellor. My first instinct was to say it didn't matter. The words froze on my tongue. Truth is, I'm learning more and more that I'm highly distrusting of men.

Honestly, I'm highly distrusting of strangers, though my friendly demeanour would have anyone believe the opposite. I just feel it's easier to ease into trust with a fellow woman. I'm sure there's some psychology about me being raised in an all female household, so that might be why I'm slightly more open towards women. I still find it incredibly sexist of me, but, at the same time, I can't help it. It's an instinct that I need to learn to overcome. Especially if I ever intend to get out there and start dating.

The point being, both myself, and this other chick decided we would both prefer to talk to women. Problem was, there was only one female counsellor available. Alex advised us that meant the second person would be waiting as much as an hour.

Of course, my brain had the snark-y come-back of, "if they have me go first, they'll be lucky if it's an hour." I didn't say it out loud, though.

When the counsellor came out, she called the other girl's name. The two of us, who had been making light conversation, looked at one another with complete confusion.

"I thought she was going first..." the other girl started.

The counsellor held up the clipboard, and, in what I felt was a needless attitude filled tone, "Well this is the name they gave me, so you're first."

"What a bitch," inner me growled. "Maybe I should have opted to talk to a guy."

On the outside, I offer a reassuring smile to the other girl. I didn't exactly have plans.

Well, I sort of did. I had asked Nick to come over Sunday night to go for sushi, and just hang out. He ended up staying the night. Thankfully, despite his best "sweet-talking", I found the strength to actually say, "No thanks. I don't feel like it tonight."

The next morning, he mentioned that he had an appointment in St Thomas. He was asking, without actually saying it, if he could come visit again. At first, I said okay.

I had a thought around noon, however, that summed up to, "Is he going to make another attempt because I said 'not tonight'? Because I really don't want to put up with that."

The fact I was at the centre when he would have been heading for his appointment was just the kick I needed to text and say, "I changed my mind. I don't think I want company tonight."

Back at the centre, the girl and counsellor disappear to the back, and I'm left alone for about 10 minutes. Then comes Alex. She said that while she was in the back, she had been trying to get in contact with a second female counsellor so that neither of us girls were waiting.

While I was waiting for her to arrive, for some reason, the memory of my encounter with that guest speaker came to mind. I remembered myself saying, "I concentrate better". Which reminded me that I do. I asked Alex if there was some paper that I could cut up into little squares to make as cranes. I explained that it helps me focus.

She found me a large, blank page, and, a little warily, provided me scissors.

And you know what? I spent the whole two hour talk with the counsellor, Ellen, folding paper cranes. I didn't cry once. Not even when touching on topics that were stressing me right now that had caused me to tear-up with Linda and Dr Adams. It was a soothing, repetitive motion to keep me balance as I talked, and listened.

I think from now on, when I go to appointments, I'm going to bring a packet of little squares with me to fold. I'll see if it makes a difference.

I now have an appointment with Ellen on Friday. She gave me a booklet to look through about different support groups I might be interested in. I'm supposed to look it over, and pick some out.

She also told me that she's going to refer me to a case manager. She said this is someone who will meet with me daily for 9 weeks to help me achieve a goal, or just help get my life together. There is a waiting list, so she told me I might not get someone until May or June, but I'm okay with that.

I was actually wondering the other day if there was such a thing as a professional that checks in on you daily to help get your life on track. Ask and you shall receive, am I right?

It seems my fears about being without supports outside of the college was unfounded. I wish Chatham had a place like this centre. It may have helped me get on track much sooner. Granted, I have no idea if I would have been able to visit it under my mother's roof.

In the end, it looks like I have steps in place to take the jump out of school at the end of the semester. It really helps quell that anxious little voice inside.

Fixing a Broken Lamp

I don't think I've ever left Dr Adams so speechless. When she first came into the room she was thanking me for coming.

"I know this must be difficult for you since I keep pushing..." but she stopped as soon as she saw my little paper cranes. I told her about my visit to the mental health clinic, and about my new technique.

We also went through the paperwork for the employment agency. I told her about how I actually bought groceries, and how I'm trying to be more sneaky about my vegetables.

For example, tomorrow I'm going to make tacos, but I'm going to cook a tomato in with the ground beef. It's not much, but I don't usually eat tomatoes. Not sure if it's the taste or texture that throws me off.

Dr Adams was pleased to hear that I had been listening to her about diet. As for exercise, I've been trying to use the stairs more often. I mean, I'm consistently winded at the same floor. Which I am proud to say isn't the first two floors, thank you very much. It makes reaching my floor all the more satisfying.

Then I told her about my rather interesting Tuesday.

Yesterday was my first full does of my new medication. By about 9 am-10am I started to feel restless. It was like I was hit with a sudden bought of energy that I didn't know what to do with. I looked around my apartment and decided I wanted to get some cleaning done.

I ended up cleaning for 2 or 3 hours. I had even done half of my dishes.

I had so much energy, I decided to repair my bedroom lamp. That thing has been broken since, I don't know, October? Maybe September. I know I hadn't lived here long when Aurora had accidentally knocked it over. The electrical in it was fine, but the neck was busted. I had put it off because I didn't have any crazy glue. It simply sat without a bulb or shade on my bedside table.

During my cleaning spree, I wondered if I could use hot glue, instead. It wouldn't hurt anything just to try it, right? To my surprise, it worked.

I don't know how, but that one light just makes the room feel more homey.

The more I got done, the better I felt. My home looks beautiful that I would even welcome a guest over. Heck, I'm expecting my mother this weekend. Of course, I wasn't thinking about that when I had started cleaning.

I think the only thing better that I could do is catch up on my classes. I suppose it is what it is. I'm not a failure. I'm just need a little more time to heal. That's what Linda meant during our last meeting when she suggested I withdraw this semester. I think, when I meet with her tomorrow morning, I'm going to see if I can make a case to still withdraw.

I know the 20th was the deadline. There's a part of me that worries I won't be able to. Thing is, when that overwhelming feeling of dread wants to crawl up my spine, I remind myself that it's going to be okay. If I can't return to school this September, it must be because I'm going to need more time to focus on my mental health.

I will return, though. If I can get employment, as I hope to, I'll save up the best I can. That way I don't have to wait until I'm off academic probation from OSAP to continue my education. I have time.

If I can withdraw, you bet your ass I'm going to use the summer to get better. Then I'm coming back in September in a stronger frame of mind. I will get this program certificate. I just have to keep trying.

Speaking of "trying again", I don't know if I mentioned that Nick visited on Sunday. Despite his attempts, I didn't sleep with him. He wanted to visit again on Monday, but I cancelled because I was at the mental health centre.

Which brings me to yesterday. As it turns out, he was in St Thomas once again. Naturally, he asked if he could visit. I did allow it, but I told him right from the start I'm not interested in anything sex related. He said he was okay with that.

He still made his excitement obvious, though. It pissed me off. I was going to sleep on the couch, again, with the excuse that I'm too hot. But then I had a thought.

"Maybe you should sleep on the couch this time," I told him while standing at the end of the bed.

There was a hint of confused surprise in his tone, "Yeah. I can do that."

That's right. Nick slept over, without getting any, AND he was on the couch while I slept peacefully in my bed.

It's been a long time coming, but I've made another hurtle. I'll be sure to make it clear to him that, when he sleeps over, the couch is where he will be staying from now on.

Unless it's a super hot night. Then I will actually want my couch because it's near my AC.

There you have it. In approximately three days I've made a come back from over a month of a low swing mood. Not bad, if I say so myself. I think it helps that I know there is support beyond the safety of the school. I'm not in this alone. I don't have to feel like I'm putting pressure on my family to be there during those hard times. Especially when they have their own issues to contend with.

I wonder what tomorrow will bring?

What Happiness Feels Like

Happy April Fool's Day to all you mischief makers. I can't say my family and I do many pranks on one another. On the rare occasions it happens, it's usually spur of the moment opportunities. We mostly just badger one another on any given day, instead.

Speaking of family, I'm waiting on my mother and sister to come visit.

I'll be glad to see Cam, but I'm super nervous about Mum coming into my home to watch a movie. During our phone conversation she was already on me about "is the apartment clean?" and "does it smell?"

I mean seriously... fuck off. I spent all of Tuesday cleaning, and felt awesome for doing it. Now I'm looking around thinking, "Mum's going to point out this and this and this." Way to add some unwanted stress to my Saturday.

Instead of focusing on it, however, I'm here writing about the last couple of days.

Thursday: Just like Dr Adams, Linda was super impressed with my progress this week. I spoke to her about options for withdrawal too. She told me that I can't withdraw since it's past the deadline. Yet, as long as I work my hardest from now until the end of the semester, she can make an argument in my favour about my mental health and change up of medication so that any classes I fail, we may be able to change to "No mark" instead.

Which is great news. I can put plenty of effort to get everything done well and on time. If it's not enough to pass, I have a possible safety net that will allow me to attend classes again.

I'm also telling myself that if the safety net falls through, maybe I'm not supposed to be going back to school in September. Maybe I'm supposed to still be working on fixing myself, and improving my life.

Linda and I then got on the topic of my paper folding. I have a thing that when I get bored of making cranes, I make paper dragons instead. They're a lot harder to do on the same scale that I do cranes. The dragon amazed her because she knew how to do cranes, but said she couldn't imagine how to make a dragon.

"It's actually super easy to do a dragon if you already know how to make a crane," I assured her. "I can teach you, if you want."

She agreed, saying she would bring paper to the art therapy group that started at 12. That way I could teach others who wanted to know, as well. Being the last group get together, there was only three students, plus Linda. One was a Vietnamese girl that I had talked to during several of the other get-togethers. For the first half hour of the group I taught those two how to fold paper dragons while the last girl painted.

I loved it. I miss teaching people. Especially teaching them something artsy. The look of joy on their faces when they held their own little dragons in their hands was magic.

Linda said that next year they should see about doing origami as one of the structured exercises. I instantly jumped on the idea saying I would love to help out on that class if they needed. This brought up the idea about having a student volunteer coordinator in future art therapy. Linda said she would bring it up during her next staff meeting, and let them know they already have a volunteer.

It really made my day.

It lead to me having a bright idea Thursday night. I wanted to add a 1/2 hour of cardio in the morning, and 1/2 hour of yoga at night as part of my new "making life better" routine.

I know I've been fighting myself on preforming routine exercises. It's not that I don't like to, it's that I never had the energy.

Thus, on Friday morning, I ventured out to find a cheap video set of cardio and yoga routines. Resulting in me doing something incredibly impulsive, but also good at the same time.

But I'll have to come back to that tonight. I just got a text saying Mum and Cam are almost here.

5 o'clock. Not a long visit, but still a good one. We went to the Saturday market. Mum didn't seem as interested in it as I was, but the three of us did get some brownies, cookies, and scons. Then we all came back to my place and watched *Fantastic Beasts and Where to Find Them.* It was much more enjoyable to watch it this time with my sister, and mother, than it was to watch with Nick.

There was a hiccup where Mum got under my skin about my apartment. I knew she would, but that doesn't make it acceptable. I asked why both of them were wearing shoes in my place. Cam covered saying she had had her hands full, and didn't think of it. Then took them off.

Mum, however, huffed, "You're floor is dirty."

"I swept just yesterday," I hissed.

"Really? Look at that," she points to the small bits of cat fur that has gathered since yesterday. "I don't want to bring that home on my socks."

Thankfully, that was the only out right dig at my home. The rest could be an easy mistake of her trying to say something, and it coming off as judgemental.

In the end, I got through it. We had a good time, and they left before one of them could really get on my nerves. Bonus is, I got my family time, and I get to sleep in my own bed tonight.

Okay, now to get into the insanity of yesterday.

I ventured out in search of the videos. My first stop was Wal-mart because I knew I had seen discount cardio videos the last time I was there. I spent a little more than intended on movies. Not all of which were work out related, but I did get my cardio routine one. There wasn't any yoga videos, though.

What I should have done is cut my loses, and just went home. I was already wet from the miserable drizzle coming down when I had to walk between bus transfers. I had also worn my heavy winter jacket to keep out the chill, but it ended up being too hot and I was sweating up a storm.

As I went out to catch the bus back, I noticed a couple places across the street. One was clearly a sports store. It turned out to be sports equipment, which you think means they would at least have yoga mats, but they didn't.

Then I crossed the parking lot to the other place. I couldn't tell from outside if it was a gym or a fitness store. I decided to have a peek, and, if it was a gym, I would cover saying I was looking for a pamphlet to compare different gyms.

They didn't have a pamphlet. They do a guided tour, tell you about the services, and only tell you the price after you show genuine interest in a membership. Or, in my case, are really good a faking interest.

I was surprised to learn that, because it was the 31st, I could be locked in at a discounted price.

To make a long story short, I joined a gym. I fucking joined a gym. Yeah, I'm still in disbelief.

I mean, okay, it's a really nice gym. The price was super good too. It actually costs me less to pay for a membership a month than to go for a single sushi dinner each month. One is a lot healthy for me, anyway.

Getting a trainer is extra. Needless to say, I was not impressed that they kept pushing about it. It took a phone call to them today for me to be able to put my foot down, but, in the end, I am not signed on to have a trainer.

Which means I am going to need to do some serious homework on proper work out routines so I can get my money's worth from this gym.

On the flip side, my membership includes free yoga classes (among others). And there's a Sauna and pool! I'm actually super excited to be going back tomorrow. I know my first concern should be school and finding work, but I have all day to do that stuff. It's nice to think I have something fun and healthy to look forward to doing for myself.

I just need to remember to not eat anything heavy more than two hours before going.

I ended up getting a complementary training session with my membership. We talked about goals, reasonable ways to obtain them, and training methods. He then wrote out three letters on his worksheet that he had been keeping notes on. The "I" representing "intensity".

I chuckled when he asked me to rate what my intensity, "I'm incredibly stubborn. If you point me to do something, I will push myself to do it until I puke."

I ended up re-tasting those words 20 minutes later. They tasted like taco wraps, and regret.

"You're a woman of your word," the trainer, said after the fact. It became a running joke for us. I think he was partially relieved because I don't think they were expecting a whole session for the free one. He was pushing me to my breaking point. 15 bar squats. 15 over head squats. 12 push-ups. 12 "Australia push-ups"; which is apparently like a chin up, but your feet are on the ground, and your body is at an angle. It was when he told me to go for as long as I could on the up and down step did my body finally say, "Really woman? Fucking stop already."

I am very impressed with myself. I haven't worked out in years. Not since I was on the junior track and field team in high school. Truly, it was exhilarating.

I ended up feeling better almost immediately after, and wanted to do more. The trainer told me that my body had clearly had enough. I was to go home, rest, and get something to eat to compensate for the calories used, and lost when I puked.

I was going to ignore his order of "give myself a day between work outs since I'm just getting back into exercise". If Mum had cancelled today, I had every intention of going back and doing the exact same work out I had done yesterday. I had plenty of time this morning.

Alas, my legs have gone on strike. I have been laughing at myself for the amount of difficulty I'm having getting on and off the toilet, for goodness sakes.

The day get's better, though.

With an exercise high running through me, I hopped the bus to the Mental Health Centre for my follow-up appointment with Ellen. I thought it was to be for 7, so I had left from the gym. It was a lot closer than anticipated, too. So, I was there just before 6:30 pm.

I found out Ellen's shift did not start until 7:30 pm. Thus, I sat in the lobby, entertaining the receptionist with my origami folding. Around 7, a nice, older lady- maybe in her early 60s- came into the centre. The receptionist was proudly showing off the crane, and the woman seemed genuinely interested.

I offered to teach her how to make a crane, if she'd like. She did. For 30 minutes we sat together first learning the crane, than talking about origami. Then I taught her the jumping frog. In fact, Ellen had come in while we were in the middle of the frog, and I asked if it was okay we finished first.

I think the paper folding had helped the older woman the same as it has helped me this past week. I can still clearly see a new spark in her blue eyes when she thanked me for teaching her.

Really, that is the sort of thing I live for.

You know, for the first time in a very long time, I have gone several consecutive days without feeling lost, anxious, or depressed. It's still there. I can hear the little nag of anxiety telling me that it's already April. I have one month to find a job, and collect a paycheck, or all these good things go away.

For right now, I'm just enjoying how good I feel. For this moment in time, I genuinely feel happy.

Healthy Changes

My body appears to be on strike. I really can't blame it because, on top of now exercising every other day, I'm dieting.

That's right. I am in the fresh hell known as a diet. Why? Because if I'm paying good money to get myself healthier at a gym, I may as well go all in.

It's not some fad kind of diet, either. I still eat what I want. I'm just making healthier alternatives, and making sure I actually eat enough calories in a day. Yes, I have an app keeping track of it for me, because I have no idea how to calorie count on my own.

In my head, I know I'm getting healthier, and the body will adjust. It's just another change I have to become accustom to.

For safety, though, I will be clearing with Dr Adams on our next meeting if I'm doing this correctly. I may know my health sciences, but I also know I am not a Doctor for a reason. It's always good to check with a heal professional when doing something like this.

Emotionally, I feel pretty good. I could do without the sugar cravings, and mild crankiness, but everything else is in check.

Speaking of crankiness, Nick got a snip of it last night. I was telling him all the stuff I just wrote above. It's an exciting new change for me.

"So, why are you suddenly going all health nut?" he asks. The way he had said, "health nut" sounded almost as if he was looking down on people for being conscious about their bodies.

Slightly irked, I tried to calmly re-explain how I came to be roped into a gym membership.

"I already know that," he cut me off. Not going to lie, I grew up getting cut off a lot. As an adult, cutting me off is a giant pet peeve. 48 hours into my new life style, and cutting me off was apparently how you make me go from irked to bitchy in four words flat.

"I mean-" he tried to finish.

I cut him off with a sharp, "I'm trying to tell you, if you would let me finish."

He tried to say some excuse. I don't fully remember what he said. I just remember hearing an edge to his tone, and it just annoyed me further.

I snapped at him again with something along the lines of, "I know what you meant, if you would stop cutting me off."

After he apologized, I waited a moment to make sure he didn't say anything else. Then I finished my explanation about the diet idea.

He did annoy me again later that night when he was showing his horn dog side. He ended up sleeping on the couch.

Thing is, I'm still rather peeved about the stupid "health nut" comment. I get that he enjoys plus size women. I think it's just another way to inflate his ego by doing something physical that I can't. Still, a little support regarding my choice to better my life would be fucking nice.

He wants to visit again tonight. I think he's not even going to be in my bed for a moment. I have no patience for any of his horn dog bull crap tonight.

I mean, I could tell him to not come over. I am considering it. I've learned enough about his attitude to know that, given the chance, he's going to try to get what he wants. Heck, I've even noticed those massages he does to be sweet tends to focus around the lower back and upper legs. That's why when he offered one when we were wondering what to do last visit, I declined.

I'm not going to lie, I'm actually happy that I'm making progress with cutting Nick back to just a friend. He keeps trying for the 'with benefits', but I am tired of this game. He has no interest in me as an individual. I'm sure when he finally realizes his advances are not going to be welcomed or tolerated, he's likely going to visit less and less.

You know what. I don't think I want him around as even a friend, anymore. I know I will get lonely, but I'm also expanding my circle with the gym, and...

Oh right! I forgot the best news I have gotten in some time. I did follow through with sending out resumes on Sunday before going to the gym. A little over 24 hours later, and I got a response. I have an interview on Friday.

It is another call centre, but there are a couple differences this time. First, it's outbound calls only. No angry customer's calling me. I'm calling someone else to sell a product.

Secondly, unlike the product of my previous call centre, this one is something I can stand by. It's actually less a product, and more a type of safety training, actually.

Lastly, it's consistent Monday to Friday hours, and I get paid commission.

I am actually really excited about this one. I feel confident about going in, because I know how call centres work. I know what they will be looking for. Best of all, I will actually get to socialize, and be paid doing it.

If all goes well in the interview, I could be starting as early as the 19th. That seems like a long time from now seeing as it's the 4th of April. Yet, it's work. I might have to borrow money from family to cover my May rent, unless I get a nice income tax return, but I'm going to make it.

God provides.

Yeah, how's this for Divine sense of humour? Sunday night, as I say my nightly prayers, I pray for work. "I really need a job by...Yesterday..." my sarcastic side supplies. But then I recover, "But I know it is all in you're timing."

Very next day from when I applied, I possibly have a job.

How awesome is that?

There is definitely a lot of good changes happening. Truly, life feels good.

Goodbye, Mr Shepard

It's still the 4th. I told Nick I didn't want to see him anymore. It was over text only because I felt that asking him to drive over so I could tell him off to his face was just rude.

Usually this turns into a big explanation, and he's trying to defend himself, and make it seem like I'm just being paranoid/crazy. I'm pretty sure that's called gaslighting. This time, though, I didn't give an explanation.

When he asked for one, all I said was, "the usual, but also I'm tired of feeling like all this is about is sex. I know you say otherwise, but your actions always say otherwise."

His response was expected, "Wow, cuz i been pressuring it? When? Just cuz i want it doesn't mean its my focus."

I told him that I was not getting into this. He can accept it or not, just so long as he respects my wishes, and leaves me alone.

"Ya sure, its your choice. Always has been," was his answer.

I wished him well, and that was that. I'm giving it a week before he texts to check in on me. Probably use some excuse. Hopefully, when that day comes, I have the strength to send him off again. I hope I can stay strong, and not text him either.

For now, I actually feel re-freed.

Carpe Diem

I got the job. We weren't even finished the entire interview and the HR lady told me I was getting the job. It's lucky my appointment was the end of the day, because it took us an hour to fill out all the questions with how many times we got off topic.

I am so happy to say, of the people I've met, friendly and happy demeanour is a common element in this workplace.

Not only that, but I had received a phone call for a second job offer just before going into the meeting.

Two job offers in one week. I have never experienced that before. I'm still amazed. Knowing that I had a second chance lined up, just in case today's interview had somehow gone wrong, made it so much easier to keep my head high as I walked into that office.

I can't believe that when Monday rolls around, I actually have to call somewhere back to *reject* a job offer. I mean, it's 1:30 am (technically the 8th of April). I've known I had the job since 4 pm, and I'm only now wrapping my head around it enough to be able to write this entry.

Wow. Simply, wow.

Everything about today was great. I didn't think it was going to since I had slept in this morning.

Admittedly, it was because I couldn't get to sleep last night. I never do on a night before an interview. I spend the entire time reciting possible answers to common interview questions. It's one of my twitches.

That extra bit of sleep was a God send that let me focus the rest of the day. It started with a meeting with Anita. I'd almost call it a visit more than a meeting because the school related stuff was covered in 10-15 minutes, tops. The rest of it was telling her about some of my plans, and just current things I'm thinking about.

I know I will likely fail at least one of my classes. But you know what? I don't feel panicked about it. School was always a choice to help keep me from being homeless, and optionless. I may not have been to many classes, but what I have learned over the last few months is even better.

I am learning to accept that my faults are not weaknesses. Strength is being kind to yourself when you make a mistake, and realizing you can over come them. That, just because I can't see a solution to a problem, doesn't mean there isn't one.

I'm reminded that hope is a powerful thing. My faith in God, myself, and others makes me brave, and wise.

I have so much more to learn, but this year has really set things in motion. For the first time in a while, I'm actually looking forward to tomorrow. I'm not frightened, or overwhelmed by the unknown. I am a little anxious that the shoe is going to drop with how much is going right, but I'm trying to fight that train of thought.

I don't feel like I'm in limbo, anymore. I have a home that isn't going to be taken from me. A place in a city where I'm out from under my mother's thumb. I have a new job that I will be starting on the 12th. I'm taking a medication that I didn't realize I had so desperately needed to help keep me from going too low in down swings.

I have connections and options for those times that my mental health starts to get the better of me.

I feel like I have a great relationship with my sister, again. I mean, we didn't even argue on her birthday this year. I'm even trying to talk her into moving up here.

Living separate from me, though. We'd probably kill each other under the same roof for more than a few hours.

I'm having a ball going to a gym I never intended to get a membership in. I am still learning how to properly keep my blood sugar regulated without falling into my sweet-tooth temptation, but I have time.

With all these changes, I felt strong enough to finally remove Nick's presence from my life. I do worry about him, but I remember he's a grown man that makes his own choices. I can't, nor should I, be responsible for his happiness. Especially when it comes at the cost of my own self worth.

Over the last couple of days without him, I've had time to really think about what I've been putting up with. The more I think about it, the more frustrated I am about letting him stay so long in my life.

I'm learning to be kinder to myself about mistakes made... Scratch that. Make it, 'being kinder to myself about *choices* made', I'm not going to regret what happened. He wasn't an awful companion, even with all the ways we clash in personality. He just had a not-so-hidden agenda, and I'm sick of dealing with it.

When I told Anita all of this, she was ecstatic for me. She was sad to here I won't be returning to school in September, but she's happy that I'm taking the time to better my physical and mental health.

"Don't worry," I told her after a giant hug. "This won't be the last you see of me. I will be back."

She laughed, "I'm going to hold you to that!" Then she went in for another big hug.

One day, I will be returning to school. I will be getting that Fine Art certificate. It doesn't matter if it takes me three or four years to save up enough money to do it, I will. I'm not failing, or quitting. I'm just postponing the goal for when I'm in a better position to fulfil it.

Anita's joy and energy allowed me to feel more up-beat when I answered the phone to that second job offer. Then, I was still all smiles as I boarded the bus to get to my interview.

The driver was the cheery of it all. He was a jolly man in his 60s. I had asked him if he knew which stop it was, and he did.

"Don't worry, we'll get you sorted out!" he cheerfully proclaimed. Loud enough for the entire bus to hear.

Slightly embarrassed, I returned to my seat at the front. I couldn't help but continue to grin, fully amused by the driver's happy-go-lucky attitude. It was infectious. To make things even better, he was whistling joyful camp tunes.

I recognized two of them as "Go tell it on a Mountain" and "The corner Grocery Store". He did others that I swear I knew the tune of, but could not place it. As I listened I was taken back to my days among Scouts Canada, St Vincent De Paul, and this other Christian Camp I went to with the church.

You know, this job has consistent hours. I should see if I can volunteer for some day camp or something to fill my evenings. I'll see how I feel once I get fully settled into this new job.

To my silent amusement, at the stop before, the driver calls out, "You're up next, Happy!"

It took a moment to realize he was referring to me. I was further surprised as I said my "thank you"s, he pipes out with, "Good luck!"

I don't remember telling him I had an interview. At the same time, I probably did while I was asking about which stop to take.

As luck would have it, his bus was the one to pick me up after the interview as well.

"How'd it go?" he smiled.

Proud as a peacock, I answered with an equally cheerful tone, "I got the job."

"Congratulations!" He then asked about when I start, and directed me to the maps holding the bus scheduling. "Man, if I wasn't on a time limit, I'd pull this bus over, and we'd all celebrate." He joked. "What do you think? Pizza sounds fantastic right about now."

Pizza sounds amazing. The first paycheck I get that has

enough wiggle room to treat myself, I'm ordering one. A small one, though. That'll be a cheat day.

With all said and done, I think it's time to close this journal up. It's a new beginning for me, so I should close this book to move on to a fresh one.

I have also been thinking of publish this. Call it another whim, or divine guidance, but it just feels like this might be why I was able to write this journal. Especially since I could never really get into writing a journal before.

I have been writing as if speaking to an imaginary audience. Maybe it's time for this piece of my journey to help others facing their fire. Or be an example to someone that is trying to understand the chaos inside their loved one's head.

If someone is reading this, seize the day.

Trust that you are much stronger than you realize. That fire can be a weight on your shoulders, but you're doing great every time you wake up. Facing another day with that inside your head makes you pretty bad ass.

Remember to enjoy the little things. Hugs, candy, or the snow falling.

On the note of little things, always hold onto hope. Just the tiniest bit can go a long way.

Be kind to yourself. We're only human, after all.

If you can bring someone a little bit of joy, do so. It doesn't have to be huge, but it might just make all the difference to them.

Most importantly, you're here for a reason. For that reason alone, you are amazing. No matter your struggles, you've got this. I believe in you.

Wishing you all the best,

Annie Burns